After You
RING THE
BELL . . .

D1487051

10 CHALLENGES
for the CANCER
SURVIVOR

BY ANNE KATZ

"This material is intended to provide general information to you. Consult your health care professional with any questions relating to a medical problem or condition."

Hygeia Media
An imprint of the Oncology Nursing Society
Pittsburgh, Pennsylvania

ONS Publications Department
Executive Director, Professional Practice and Programs:
Elizabeth M. Wertz Evans, RN, MPM, CPHQ, CPHIMS, FACMPE
Publisher and Director of Publications: Barbara Sigler, RN, MNEd
Managing Editor: Lisa M. George, BA
Technical Content Editor: Angela D. Klimaszewski, RN, MSN
Staff Editor II: Amy Nicoletti, BA
Copy Editor: Laura Pinchot, BA
Graphic Designer: Dany Sjoen

Library of Congress Cataloging-in-Publication Data

Katz, Anne (Anne Jennifer), 1958-
  After you ring the bell : 10 challenges for the cancer survivor / by Anne Katz.
    p. cm.
  Includes bibliographical references.
  ISBN 978-1-935864-15-8 (alk. paper)
  1. Cancer--Popular works. 2. Cancer--Patients--Popular works. I. Title.
  RC263.K275 2011
  616.99'4--dc23

                                                                        2011032514

Publisher's Note

This book is published by the Oncology Nursing Society (ONS). ONS neither represents nor guarantees that the practices described herein will, if followed, ensure safe and effective patient care. The recommendations contained in this book reflect ONS's judgment regarding the state of general knowledge and practice in the field as of the date of publication. The recommendations may not be appropriate for use in all circumstances. Those who use this book should make their own determinations regarding specific safe and appropriate patient-care practices, taking into account the personnel, equipment, and practices available at the hospital or other facility at which they are located. The editors and publisher cannot be held responsible for any liability incurred as a consequence from the use or application of any of the contents of this book. Figures and tables are used as examples only. They are not meant to be all-inclusive, nor do they represent endorsement of any particular institution by ONS. Mention of specific products and opinions related to those products do not indicate or imply endorsement by ONS. Web sites mentioned are provided for information only; the hosts are responsible for their own content and availability. Unless otherwise indicated, dollar amounts reflect U.S. dollars.

ONS publications are originally published in English. Publishers wishing to translate ONS publications must contact ONS about licensing arrangements. ONS publications cannot be translated without obtaining written permission from ONS. (Individual tables and figures that are reprinted or adapted require additional permission from the original source.) Because translations from English may not always be accurate or precise, ONS disclaims any responsibility for inaccuracies in words or meaning that may occur as a result of the translation. Readers relying on precise information should check the original English version.

Printed in the United States of America

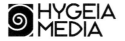

An imprint of the Oncology Nursing Society

Words and words
Lines and lines
Pages and pages
Again and again
for Alan

Disclosure

Editors and authors of books and guidelines provided by the Oncology Nursing Society are expected to disclose to the readers any significant financial interest or other relationships with the manufacturer(s) of any commercial products.

A vested interest may be considered to exist if a contributor is affiliated with or has a financial interest in commercial organizations that may have a direct or indirect interest in the subject matter. A "financial interest" may include, but is not limited to, being a shareholder in the organization; being an employee of the commercial organization; serving on an organization's speakers bureau; or receiving research from the organization. An "affiliation" may be holding a position on an advisory board or some other role of benefit to the commercial organization. Vested interest statements appear in the front matter for each publication.

Contributors are expected to disclose any unlabeled or investigational use of products discussed in their content. This information is acknowledged solely for the information of the readers.

The author provided the following disclosure and vested interest information:

Anne Katz, RN, PhD: AstraZeneca, honoraria, other remuneration

TABLE OF CONTENTS

Chapter 1. Introduction..1
Defining Cancer Survivorship.......................................1
Transitioning From Active Treatment 4
Being "Cancer Free" 6
So What Happens Next? 8
Ring That Bell!...11

Chapter 2. Sometimes a Cough Is Just a Cough............13
How Does This Fear Manifest Itself?............................14
What Else Plays a Role in Fear of Recurrence? 17
So What Can You Do to Manage the Fear? 19
Take-Home Messages 31

Chapter 3. Battling the Blues....................................33
What Is Depression?...33
Depression and Cancer 35
Getting Help for Depression 44
Take-Home Messages 52

Chapter 4. Walking Through Mud.............................53
What Does This Fatigue Feel Like? 54
What Plays a Role in This Fatigue? 56
What Can Be Done About It? 59
Take-Home Messages 69

Chapter 5. Moving Right Along 71
What About Nutrition? 71
How Does Exercise Help?..78

The Importance of Quitting Smoking 84
Alcohol 87
Sun Protection 87
Vitamin and Mineral Supplements 88
Why Is It Important to Make Lifestyle Changes? 89
Take-Home Messages 90

Chapter 6. On High Alert 93
How Do You Remember the Treatments? 93
What Is a Survivorship Care Plan? 96
What Does the Survivorship Care Plan Look Like? 101
Childhood Cancer Survivors 104
Adult Cancer Survivors 107
Take-Home Messages 108

Chapter 7. Protection for Life 109
What Are Common Long-Term and Late Effects
    of Treatment? 111
How Can These Late Effects Be Prevented? 121
Which Late Effects Can Be Minimized or Prevented? 121
Take-Home Messages 124

Chapter 8. In a Fog 127
What Causes Cancer-Related Cognitive Changes? 129
What Do Cancer-Related Cognitive Changes Look
    and Feel Like? 130
Are There Tests to Find Cognitive Changes? 134
What Treatments Can Help With Cognitive Changes? 136
Alternatives to Medication 140
Take-Home Messages 142

Chapter 9. Being a Part of It All 145
Why Go Back to Work? 146
What Makes Going Back to Work Easier? 149
What Are the Pitfalls to Look Out For? 151
When Things Go Bad 154
Making Going Back to Work, Work 157
Take-Home Messages 159

Chapter 10. Up Close and Personal 161
What Are the Most Common Sexual Problems After
    Treatment? 162

Talking About It 167
What Can Help With Sexual Problems? 170
What Can Get in the Way of Getting Help? 177
What If You're Single? 179
Take-Home Messages 180

Chapter 11. Empty Nests 183
How Does Cancer Affect Male Fertility? 184
How Does Cancer Affect Female Fertility? 185
Talking About Fertility After Cancer 186
What Fertility Preservation Options Are There? 188
What Do Patients With Cancer Need to Know About Fertility
    After Cancer? 191
Effects of Infertility on Couples and Individuals 194
Take-Home Messages 197

Chapter 12. Resources 199
Web Sites 199
Books 199
Mindfulness-Based Stress Reduction 201
Sensual Massage and Sensate Focus Exercises 201
Fertility Organizations 205

Bibliography 207

Index 213

CHAPTER 1

INTRODUCTION

C ancer survivors are a growing population. The latest estimate is that almost 12 million Americans, almost 4% of the total population, are living after a cancer diagnosis. About 65% of adults diagnosed with cancer are alive five years after their diagnosis, and more than one million survivors are alive 25 years or more after diagnosis. This is something to celebrate, so if you are one of those 12 million, take a moment and congratulate yourself on your membership in this amazing group. If you are a family member of someone with cancer, pat yourself on the back too. As you will see throughout this book, cancer survivorship includes family and friends who provide the essential support, love, and encouragement to those with cancer, and they couldn't do it without you. If you are a healthcare provider, you have likely played an important role in treating and caring for many survivors from the beginning of their cancer journey.

DEFINING CANCER SURVIVORSHIP

So who is a cancer survivor? No mention of cancer survivorship existed in the medical and nursing literature until the

1980s. In 1985, cancer survivor and physician Fitzhugh Mullan described three "seasons" of survival in a landmark article in the prestigious *New England Journal of Medicine*. The first season is that of *acute survival*, which begins with diagnosis and continues to the end of active treatment. The second season, *extended survival*, begins at the end of treatment and continues through the period of disease remission and is seen as a period of watchful waiting. The third season is described as *permanent survival* or *cure*.

These seasons of survival have been further elaborated upon. A season of *transitional cancer survivorship* is suggested to occur when the person moves from the period of active treatment to one of careful observation and when adaptation to the physical, emotional, and social changes happens. Extended survivorship (the second season) is now seen to embrace three groups of survivors: those who are alive and living with cancer but require ongoing treatment for recurrence or advanced disease, those in complete remission who require ongoing treatment, or those in complete remission with a favorable prognosis. Some of the survivors in this second season will live long lives, whereas others will experience progression of their disease. Permanent survival is now thought of as comprising four subgroups:

- Those who are cancer free but not free of cancer, as their lives are irrevocably changed
- Those who are cancer free but live with significant challenges physically, emotionally, financially, legally, and socially
- Those who go on to develop secondary cancers unrelated to their primary cancer
- Those who develop cancers secondary to their treatments.

But much has changed since the 1980s when Mullan described his view of cancer survivorship. Many cancers, such as prostate and breast, are now diagnosed at a relatively early age. Treatments have improved, and as a result, many more people are living past diagnosis and treatment. The side effects of some treatments are now better controlled and even prevented, allowing for a reduction in the numbers of people dying from these effects. New and emerging therapies allow some cancers to be treated effectively where before there was little hope. Bone marrow and stem cell transplantation has evolved dramatically, providing greater hope and even remission or cure for cancers that were immediately lethal in years past. However, these changes have downsides, too: More survivors live long enough after initial diagnosis and treatment to develop secondary cancers related to their initial treatment or new cancers. And many cancer survivors now live long enough to experience the effects of aging that are compounded by late effects from treatment.

Today cancer survivorship has many different definitions, and researchers and oncology care providers often don't agree on the "best" or "most accurate" definition. The Office of Cancer Survivorship at the National Cancer Institute considers cancer survivorship to start at the time of diagnosis and to continue for the balance of the person's life. They include family, friends, and caregivers as survivors too because they are also affected by the diagnosis. In 2004, the President's Cancer Panel defined cancer survivorship this way:

> Among healthcare professionals, people with a cancer history, and the public, views differ as to when a person with cancer becomes a survivor. Many consider a person to be a survivor from the moment of di-

agnosis; in recent years this view has become increasingly prevalent. Some, however, think that a person with a cancer diagnosis cannot be considered a survivor until he or she completes initial treatment. Others believe a person with cancer can be considered a survivor if he or she lives five years beyond diagnosis. Still others believe survivorship begins at some other point after diagnosis and treatment, and some reject the term "survivor" entirely, preferring to think of people with a cancer history as fighters, "thrivers," champions, patients, or simply as individuals who have had a life-threatening disease. A considerable number of people with a cancer history maintain that they will have survived cancer if they die from another cause.

Do any of these definitions matter? Perhaps to policy makers and researchers who have to plan programs and studies, knowing who can access the services or studies is important. But to the person who has been diagnosed with cancer, life after cancer does not have to fit into certain parameters. For people living with cancer and its aftermath, life has changed. Life with cancer has both positive and negative aspects, and although everyone's experience is unique, some experiences seem to be universal.

TRANSITIONING FROM ACTIVE TREATMENT

Life during treatment is a very controlled one; you attend appointments for chemotherapy or radiation daily or a couple of times a week or every month. Your healthcare providers tell you what to do and where to be. They are efficient and caring, and they make you feel important and cared for. In many ways, you are controlled by your treatment. As human beings, we like to think we are in control. Cancer has probably taught you that, in fact, we have very little control. You may have done everything right before the cancer—you ate healthily and exercised and didn't smoke or drink to excess—and yet you still got cancer!

And then, once treatment ends, that controlled environment is no longer a part of your every day or week. You are on your own, picking up the pieces of your life after a significant interruption. Your family and friends may celebrate this milestone—your treatment is over, you can get back to living your old life, and things will be back to normal. Many myths are associated with the end of treatment, such as the following.

- The end of treatment is a time to celebrate and forget the cancer.
- Recovery should occur soon after treatment ends.
- You should quickly go back to your "old" self.
- You don't need support after treatment is over.

What?! Sure you can celebrate the end of treatment, but many people are just too sick and tired to do much besides rest and try to figure out what just happened. And you may never be able to forget what you have gone through. Recovery can take many months, and there is no timetable for feeling better or stronger or more energized. You may never go back to the way you were; physical and emotional changes may make you better than you were before, stronger and wiser but not the same. And we all need support, perhaps even more so when treatment ends.

So how do you make the transition from active treatment to recovery and survivorship? It may be helpful to think of this transition as one that involves three stages: (a) endings, (b) a neutral zone, and eventually (c) a new beginning. When treatment ends, so too do the intense relationships you had with your oncology care providers and the safety they represent. You have to give up being the patient. Although it was a forced and reluctant role, it provided one with attention, reassurance, and support. Leaving that behind can be frightening and lonely. When treatment ends, you move into what has been called the *neutral zone*, which is characterized by feelings of chaos, loss, and confusion. Where are you? What comes next? For many, a new beginning emerges in its own time, when the survivor has resolved the issues from the end of treatment and the questions from the neutral zone.

Transitioning from active treatment is stressful. Not only have you lost the intense contacts and monitoring of your health, but now that treatment is over, you may begin to worry about the cancer coming back. You may not be clear on what comes next, how your health will be monitored, and whether you will recognize signs of things going wrong or will know what to do if that happens. You may be feeling at your very worst as the side effects of chemotherapy or radiation are at their most intense. And you may not know how you are going to go back to being what you were before—a parent, a family member, a worker, a "normal" person.

BEING "CANCER FREE"

What does it mean to be *cancer free*? Are you ever cancer free? Some would suggest that for the person who has had cancer, though there may be no evidence of the disease after treatment, one is never free of the cancer. Not only are there lingering long-term effects, such as fatigue and perhaps changes to both body image and functioning, but there also may be abiding worry about the cancer coming back.

We know that cancer survivors are resilient and can teach the rest of us important lessons about strength and courage and humor. Many survivors say that cancer changed their lives for the better, that ironically something that most of us fear can have a silver lining. Many cancer survivors come through treatment with a sense of mastery and self-esteem. They have faced something terrible and traumatic and yet have grown emotionally and spiritually and have found meaning in their lives from the experience.

Cancer survivors commonly report improved relationships with family and friends and experiencing a deeper love for their partner or spouse and close family members. They often find that they want to invest more time and energy in these relationships, which in turn deepens and improves the relationships even more. Cancer survivors also report that they cope better with whatever life throws at them; they are more likely to accept things as they come and to cope more effectively with stress. And the cancer experience tends to imbue survivors with greater compassion for others and a better outlook on life.

But some do not cope with the cancer or adapt to the new reality of life after cancer. Many factors can negatively affect what happens after cancer. These include more advanced disease, less social support, poor relationships with oncology care providers, rigid coping styles, being a natural pessimist and having a helpless and hopeless outlook on life, and being in a difficult spousal or partner relationship.

SO WHAT HAPPENS NEXT?

The answer to this important question, in part, lies in the rest of the book. At least I hope it does! In the next 10 chapters of this book, you will read about 10 important features of cancer survivorship. Why 10? Why *these* 10? For the past 10 years in my role as a sexuality counselor in a large cancer center in Canada, I have worked with cancer survivors experiencing sexual difficulties. In working with these cancer survivors and their partners and spouses, I became increasingly interested in the challenges they face in their daily lives, outside of their sexual difficulties. I began to read about this phenomenon called *cancer survivorship,* and as I read and thought and digested the information I was reading, I saw some trends emerge from my readings. It became apparent to me that cancer survivors face 10 key issues, and in the following chapters, I describe these challenges and what to do about them.

Chapter 2. Sometimes a Cough Is Just a Cough: The number-one fear of most cancer survivors is of the cancer coming back. Every ache and pain, cough, or sneeze sends the survivor into panic mode: Is the cancer back? This chapter will address this fear of recurrence, which for some survivors can be overwhelming. It can also be an issue for loved ones who may watch the survivor like hawks, terrified that it will all happen again. This chapter will provide strategies to help survivors and their loved ones cope with this fear, helping to keep it in balance while maintaining vigilance.

Chapter 3. Battling the Blues: Many cancer survivors find that after all the activity and attention during the treatment phase, they are depressed. Often their family and friends do not understand why this is happening and tell the survivor to just be happy to be alive. Depression is common among cancer survivors and has been linked to a risk of recurrence. This chapter will address this important topic with tips on how to manage depression with medication and other nonprescription interventions.

Chapter 4. Walking Through Mud: Cancer survivors often assume that once treatment is over, they will feel "normal" again. They may be surprised when side effects linger for a long time. Fatigue is one contributor to feeling this way. Many factors affect energy levels, and these will be described in this chapter along with suggestions to combat them.

Chapter 5. Moving Right Along: Treatment for cancer can ravage the body, and it is important to eat well and exercise to regain strength and heal the body. But these kinds of lifestyle changes are very difficult to make and sustain. How do you find the motivation to exercise when all you want to do is rest? With all the hype about what foods are good to eat and what can "prevent" cancer, what is the survivor to do? This chapter will provide evidence-based answers to these questions and more.

Chapter 6. On High Alert: Cancer survivors must monitor their health, especially for recurrence or secondary cancers. But how do you know what to look for? When should you see your oncologist, and when should you schedule tests and investigations? What should you tell other healthcare providers who are not part of the cancer team? One way of keeping all this straight is to have a survivorship care plan, a carefully laid out document of what to look for, what tests to have, and how often, as well as a detailed description of the treatments you received.

Chapter 7. Protection for Life: Many of the treatments for cancer result in long-term complications or side effects. Examples of this include weak bones (osteoporosis), hot flashes, and increased risk for the development of diabetes. This chapter will describe the most common late and long-term side effects and will offer suggestions for early recognition as well as coping.

Chapter 8. In a Fog: Cancer-related cognitive changes (called *chemobrain* in the past) are one of the more significant and scary challenges of life after cancer. These changes can interfere with memory, language, and other activities involving the brain. These changes are not only related to chemotherapy but also may be the result of radiation or the diagnosis itself. This chapter will describe and explain this frightening phenomenon and make suggestions for how to cope with these changes, for both survivors and their loved ones.

Chapter 9. Being a Part of It All: Many cancer survivors want to or have to go back to work after treatment, but this is not always easy. Changes to tasks and responsibilities may have to be made. This chapter will highlight some of the challenges and opportunities in creating a back-to-work plan for cancer survivors.

Chapter 10. Up Close and Personal: Sexual and relationship changes are a common challenge after cancer treatment. After the many months of treatment, it is usually in the survivor-ship phase of the cancer trajectory that couples start to think about being sexual again. All cancer treatments affect sexuality in some way, and it often is difficult to ask for help. This chapter will provide strategies to address this sensitive topic with partners and healthcare providers.

Chapter 11. Empty Nests: Many cancer survivors have not started or completed childbearing when the diagnosis of cancer is made. This can present some significant challenges. Couples who are dealing with infertility are twice as likely to be depressed than those who are able to conceive easily. A great deal of misinformation and inaccurate promises exist about fertility treatments. This chapter will provide the latest evidence about fertility after cancer treatment in a caring and compassionate manner.

Chapter 12. Resources: This chapter provides print and Web-based resources for information about life after cancer. It also contains detailed explanations of some of the techniques mentioned in the other chapters of the book.

Bibliography: Here you will find some selected papers and books that I have used in the research for this book. They are mostly academic papers that can be found through college and university libraries, online, or even at your local public library.

RING THAT BELL!

Many cancer centers have a bell for patients to ring the day they have their last treatment. The bell signals to staff and other patients that someone has ended treatment, that someone has reached a milestone in the cancer journey that at one time seemed to be just a distant dream. For some, ringing the bell means the beginning of cancer survivorship, a new phase in the journey, a passage from patient to something else.

But what does it mean to be a cancer survivor? Are your worries over? Will side effects of treatment magically disappear and life go back to what it was before? Take a deep breath, turn the page, and start to read. Your journey is not over—there is more to learn and experience. Bon voyage!

CHAPTER 2

SOMETIMES A COUGH IS JUST A COUGH

Fear of recurrence has been cited as one of the sentinel experiences of cancer survivorship. During the time of treatment, most people with cancer can only think about getting through, getting done, surviving. But treatment comes to an end, and you are done, you got through, you are a survivor. Then a thought pops into your head: What if the cancer comes back? What will I do? Could I possibly go through all of this again?

The fear may be of the same cancer coming back or cancer developing in another part of the body. It is very common and may in fact be universal in that *all* cancer survivors have some element of this fear. It can extend far beyond the end of the treatment phase, and often healthcare providers do not address it. This fear of recurrence contributes greatly to psychological distress and has a negative impact on quality of life and energy. Family members are prone to these same fears and may even be more worried than the survivors themselves. Being prepared for this fear and understanding how to manage it is essential for survivors and their loved ones.

HOW DOES THIS FEAR MANIFEST ITSELF?

Fear of recurrence is not a simple thing to understand. It has many different facets or elements. It is not purely emotional, and so positive thinking or other simplistic solutions do not help cancer survivors control their fear. It has been suggested that fear of recurrence is related to cues or triggers that may be internal or external.

Internal cues are physical sensations such as a sudden pain or a new sensation somewhere in the body, like the sudden onset of a cough. The survivors sometimes then interpret these sensations as being related to the original cancer or as a sign that the cancer has spread. Interpretation of physical symptoms is an area of high uncertainty. Many survivors try to find an explanation for new physical sensations to reduce their fear. In recent years, the issue of late effects of cancer treatment has become widely recognized in the medical world. However, cancer survivors may not be well informed about these late effects. They may think that a new symptom is a recurrence of the cancer, when in fact it is a side effect of the original treatment occurring many months or years later.

Mary is 60 years old and was diagnosed with breast cancer almost 8 years ago. As a single mother of two teenage sons, she was unable to take much time off work at the time and pushed herself to get back to normal as soon as possible. Her insurance didn't allow her to have reconstructive surgery, and so she has lived with a large mastectomy scar on her left chest wall all these years. She was very happy when after five years the oncologist told her that she didn't need to be seen at the cancer center any longer. She continues to go for a yearly mammogram on the other breast. Ever since her surgery, the skin around the mastectomy scar has been numb and at times itchy. But she was shocked when last week she felt a burning sensation over the scar, and her first thought was that the cancer was back. She called her family doctor in a panic and was annoyed when she could only get an appointment for the next week. What if it was cancer? Surely waiting a week to see the doctor was too long?

External cues also play a role. *External cues* are events that remind the person of the cancer experience, such as a program on TV or an article in a magazine about the same kind of cancer, or hearing about a celebrity diagnosed with cancer. These events bring on fears that the cancer is back or that another cancer has developed somewhere. In response to these cues, some cancer survivors respond in a negative way. They may become hypervigilant, seeking out confirmation or negation of their symptoms by physical examination of themselves or constant checking on the Internet for evidence to support or refute their fears. They may seek out medical care from a variety of care providers, either not believing what they are told or trying to find someone who will confirm their worst fears even if they are unfounded. Others may avoid routine medical care, fearing that they will hear that the cancer has returned and dealing with their anxiety through avoidance.

While she waits for her appointment the next week, Mary finds that she is constantly touching the scar, trying to figure out if the burning sensation is getting better or worse. Her boys have lives of their own and she is alone most of the time when at home; she finds herself running her fingers over the smooth, white scar as she watches TV. Is there a change? Did it always feel so hard? Is the scar thicker? All of these questions cause her heart to race and palms to sweat.

Another important part of the fear of cancer is the presence of intrusive thoughts. These are thoughts, always negative, that seem to just pop into your head without any trigger or cue. These thoughts tend to be future oriented, are most often about the cancer, and are experienced in both verbal and image forms. For example, you may see yourself walking into the cancer center again, you may even recognize the smell from memory, and your heart starts to beat faster and you feel sick to your stomach at what lies ahead. You may say to yourself, "Not again; how am I going to do this all over?" and you feel your anxiety level shoot upward.

Intrusive thoughts can be either an obsession or a worry. They differ in degree and outcome; obsessions tend to be experienced as more negative and intrusive. They are difficult to control and tend to cause high levels of distress and anxiety. Worries are also negative and unwanted, but they often are an attempt to solve a problem whose outcome is not certain and where one or more negative outcomes are possible. They also occur more frequently than obsessions and tend to last longer. Worries usually are experienced as verbal

thoughts and have more easily identifiable triggers than obsessions.

> *Mary finds herself thinking about the pain constantly while at work. She has little privacy on the floor of the department store where she has worked for the past 15 years, but in her mind she plays out the various scenarios: She imagines herself sitting in the doctor's waiting room, her hand itching to once again touch the scar and assess the pain. Then she sees herself in the examination room, the doctor placing his cold hands over the scar and pressing, pushing, prodding. She hears the doctor say, "I think I'd like you to have more tests, Mary," and she feels the tears prick behind her eyes. Then she imagines the doctor examining her, but this time Dr. Wilson tells her that there is nothing to worry about, and it's just the nerves growing even after all this time. Her mood changes instantly, but then doubt overcomes her again. She imagines having to undergo chemotherapy and radiation, and she feels sick to her stomach.*

WHAT ELSE PLAYS A ROLE IN
FEAR OF RECURRENCE?

Personal factors that affect the fear of recurrence include being younger at the time of diagnosis, having more education, and being female. All of these factors are associated with higher levels of anxiety about recurrence. Older survivors with cancer may assume that symptoms such as fatigue or joint stiffness are related to aging and not recurrence of the cancer. This can be both a positive and negative factor. It is positive when the assumption is that a symptom is related to aging and not anything to get upset about. But it can be negative in that some symptoms may be ignored and not reported to a healthcare provider. Being closer to the time of diagnosis also results in greater fear of recurrence. Physical symptoms such as fatigue also increase these fears. African American survivors appear to have fewer fears and identify fewer triggers for these fears than Caucasian survivors.

> *Mary considers telling her sons about this but then shakes her head. Billy, her oldest, is out of work, and she thinks he is drinking too much. He lives four blocks away but he doesn't like her to drop in without an invitation. Danny is her favorite son, although she wouldn't admit that out loud. But he lives in another state, and she sees him only once or twice a year at most. He recently moved in with his girlfriend, Lisa, and Mary doesn't like her all that much. They had only met once and it did not go well. Lisa comes from a rich family and seemed to be uncomfortable in Mary's small apartment with its modest furniture that is showing its age.*

Life stressors affect fear of recurrence in direct and indirect ways. When there is other stress in the family, both the cancer survivor and the family members report negative feelings and increased anxiety. It is clear that a great deal of interdependence exists between the cancer survivor's fears and those of family members; fear breeds fear and affects adjustment to life after cancer. Greater family support and resiliency tends to decrease the fear of recurrence, perhaps by allowing for a more realistic appraisal of the situation and reaching out for help with worries. Cancer survivors and their family members who attach positive meaning to the cancer experience appear to have less fear of recurrence.

SO WHAT CAN YOU DO TO MANAGE THE FEAR?

You can manage the fear of recurrence in a variety of ways. Being in **denial** is one way of coping, although this is ultimately not an effective coping mechanism. You can find ways to stop thinking about the cancer. Some people do this by self-medicating with drugs or alcohol, by working long hours, or indulging in other distractions. Denial is hard to maintain for a long time, and eventually you have to face your fears. Or someone in your family will force you to face them by reminding you of an upcoming appointment for follow-up care or asking repeatedly how you are and if you think about the cancer.

Mary continues to worry about the pain but does nothing to help herself. She is not sleeping well, and when she looks in the mirror, she looks years older than her age. She has dark circles under her eyes and her mouth is pinched. She finds herself thinking about what will happen next, and most of her thoughts are about her relationship with her sons and how they will react when she dies. These thoughts upset her, and she has started to leave the light on in her bedroom at night. Lying in the dark makes her very afraid, and she often wonders if that is what being dead feels like. Most days all she can do is get up, go to work, and then come home and go directly to bed. She doesn't even check the answering machine on her phone, and it feels like months since she last spoke to Billy or Danny.

It is also important to **identify exactly what it is you are afraid of**. Are you afraid of having to go through treatment again? Or is it the uncertainty about the future that is making you afraid? Are you afraid that if the cancer recurs, you think you will die? Do you think that a recurrence of the cancer means that somehow you have failed? These are some of the common stressors that cancer survivors experience. There are rational answers to all these questions, but fear is not a rational thing. It sometimes helps to write down your fears on a piece of paper. Just writing them down can take away some of their power. It also helps to "see" your feelings in words. This can help you to realize that in many ways, fears are just words, and by naming them, you can start to take some control over them.

If you find that intrusive thoughts and worries or obsessions are interfering with your daily life or ability to cope, there are some things you can do to help with that. First, note when you have these thoughts and if anything triggers them. You can write in a **diary** or even just a plain notebook. Does knowing that you have a follow-up appointment with your oncologist trigger these intrusive thoughts? What happens to you when these thoughts occur? Does your heart start to pound and your palms get sweaty? Do you feel short of breath or sick to your stomach? How intense were these feelings, and what did you do about them, if anything? Did you take some slow, deep breaths, or did you distract yourself by turning on the TV or going for a walk? How helpful was that? What would you do differently the next time it happens? By writing this down, you will notice similarities between these occurrences. You will also then know what to do about it the next time or what else you can try to control your response to the intrusive thoughts.

One way to control these thoughts is to **refocus** them. For example, if you know you have an appointment with the oncologist coming up and a negative and fear-provoking thought comes into your head—"What will I do if the cancer comes back?"—consciously change that thought. Instead of focusing on the negative emotion of the cancer coming back, you replace the thought with a more rational and calming thought: "I have been feeling well, and this is a routine follow-up appointment." This may feel awkward and strained at first, but with time it will become more natural. Instead of experiencing the physical signs of anxiety (the raised heart rate and breathlessness), you will be able to calm both your mental and physical reactions to these thoughts and remain in control of your responses.

Something that can really help you to relax and calm yourself is **progressive muscle relaxation**. This is a simple technique to learn and one that can be done at any time you feel stressed and tense and before you go to bed to help you fall asleep. An important part of learning this technique is being able to concentrate on the sensations in your muscles when they are tense and when they are relaxed.

Begin this exercise by sitting down comfortably in a chair. Breathe in and out slowly and deeply. Then, starting with your feet, tense the muscles tightly and hold for five seconds. Pay attention to what this feels like, and then relax the muscles as you breathe out. Think about what those relaxed muscles feel like. Use your abdominal muscles to pull the air into your lungs and then to blow it out. Concentrate on the sensation of tense muscles and then relaxed muscles. After you have tensed and relaxed the muscles of your feet, do the same for the muscles of your calves, and then your thighs, and then move up your body (stomach, buttocks, back, shoulders, arms, hands, neck, face, and head), remembering to breathe in and out as you tense and relax. Once you have done this over your whole body, allow a feeling of complete relaxation to move down your body as you slowly and deeply breathe in and out. Concentrate on this feeling and store it in your memory. The aim is to be able to achieve that feeling of relaxation again when you need it to calm yourself. When you first learn how to do this, you have to consciously tense your muscles and then relax them. Over time you will learn to relax the muscles without having to first tense them.

It really helps to practice this exercise three to four times a week, taking about 15 minutes to move through the various parts of your body. One day you will find that you can relax your body just by thinking about being relaxed. You may find it helpful to note your level of tension before and after each session; you will see that over time you are more relaxed when you start and even more relaxed after the exercise. You can do this while sitting in a waiting room before a medical appointment, while your blood is being drawn for tests, or any time you feel anxious or afraid.

Deep breathing can help with muscle relaxation, as well as with your everyday activities. Breathing may seem to be an automatic function, but many of us breathe using the muscles of our shoulders and chest, which causes shallow breathing. When you are anxious, you tend to take shallow breaths quite rapidly. This may even make you feel weak and faint. By breathing with your abdominal muscles, you draw more air into your lungs more slowly. This is better for you and promotes relaxation.

How do you breathe with your abdominal muscles? Start by placing the palm of your hand over your belly button. Now push your hand away using your stomach muscles and feel the air enter your lungs as the muscles push outward. Now pull your hand back as you exhale, pushing the air out of your lungs with those same muscles. You should breathe like this when you do your progressive muscle exercises. It feels quite strange at first, which is proof in itself of how familiar it feels to breathe from our shoulders and chest. It takes practice to always breathe like this, but you will notice that as it becomes your new normal way of breathing, you will feel more relaxed.

Another useful technique to control fear is **mindfulness-based stress reduction** (MBSR). This technique comes from the disciplines of meditation and yoga and has been used very successfully in the treatment of a number of illnesses, including cancer. It is not a religious practice and does not require any kind of belief, just practice and more practice. The aim of MBSR is to keep yourself focused on the moment without the distractions of the past or the future. Relaxation may result from mindfulness; however, it is not the aim of this technique.

Being focused on the moment is not as easy as it sounds because, as humans, we tend to be future oriented and attached to the memories of our past.

MBSR is usually learned in a series of classes that take place over 6–10 weeks with homework assignments to be done between classes. Many hospitals and cancer centers offer classes in MBSR to help patients and survivors control anxiety and feelings of helplessness as they journey through the different parts of the cancer experience. CDs can also be purchased that can help you learn this technique if no classes are in your area. You need to practice this technique six days a week for 15–45 minutes each session.

Four different kinds of mindfulness practice exist:
• Awareness of sensation
• Sitting meditation
• Body scan
• Mindful movement.

In the first of these, awareness of sensation, the first thing you do is learn what the sensation of breathing feels like. Sit comfortably in a chair, and, very similar to the previous section on deep breathing, concentrate on the sensation of the air entering and leaving your lungs as you take slow, deep breaths. This will allow you to relax. You should be able to elicit this feeling of relaxation whenever you need it, simply by sitting quietly and breathing.

Once you have mastered the awareness of sensation, it is time to move on to sitting meditation. In this activity, you focus on a single physical sensation, and by giving it your full attention, you alter it. For example, if you have a backache, by focusing intently on the pain in your back, you can influence how you feel about the pain. You will notice the quality of the pain (dull, aching, sharp, coming and going), and your focus on the pain itself will block out the thoughts you have about the pain (why am I in pain, what does it mean, is it related to the cancer). You can apply the same activity to feelings: concentrate on what you are feeling, and see that your focus will block other negative thoughts and feelings.

The third form of MBSR is the body scan, which is quite similar to the progressive muscle relaxation technique described earlier. But this time, you move from your head to your feet, slowly going over the different parts of your body and focusing on how each part feels. This exercise will put you in touch with your body in a very deliberate way, and you will learn about how your body really feels—where it is tense, where it is relaxed, where you feel hunger, where you feel pain—and then be able to address those areas in a constructive manner.

The final kind of MBSR is mindful movement, which is often taught in the form of yoga. Learning about the strength and flexibility of the body is a powerful tool to help with physical and emotional healing. Despite the challenges of treatment, the body still supports us in our daily lives, and even with limitations, there is much to be grateful for.

Most of us are not mindful in our daily activities. We rush through our day, thinking about what we have to do or remember, or focusing on what happened last night or last week. We miss so many opportunities to be grateful about the many moments that bring joy and healing. Think about your walk to the corner store or to work or to the mailbox today. Did you breathe deeply and smell the smells of the season? Did you feel the sun on your back or the chill of the winter wind? Did you appreciate the sensation of your feet moving you along? Most of us rush through these everyday activities, not aware of the sights, sounds, smells, and sensations that flow over our bodies every second. By being in the moment and appreciating those sights, sounds, smells, and sensations, we can truly be alive, aware, and appreciative. But, instead, we think about what we have to do and what we have left behind. Our shoulders tense and we take shallow breaths, and a pleasurable activity becomes something strained and unpleasant.

MBSR allows cancer survivors to let go of the painful memories of diagnosis and treatment and the fear and uncertainty of the future. By focusing on the present, being in the moment, you can fully LIVE the here and now, unencumbered by memory or anticipation. Even if you experience pain in the moment, giving it your full attention allows it to be just what it is, nothing more. This can help you to cope with it and not make it something more or worse than it is.

Doing some kind of **exercise** can also be helpful. Exercise is a form of distraction that produces endorphins, hormones that naturally raise our mood and alleviate depression. You will read over and over in this book about the many benefits of exercise. Moving our bodies can make us appreciative of the good things that our bodies can do. This can offset the negative feelings that we may have after cancer, when the body is sometimes seen as having let us down. Getting exercise in a group setting can also forge new friendships and make us feel normal, like everyone else.

Mary kept the appointment with her family doctor, and he told her it was nothing to worry about. She didn't believe him and continued to struggle with sleep-less nights and worry-filled days. A couple of weeks lat-er, Mary is home when the phone rings. She doesn't even try to get out of bed to answer, even though it is just past six o'clock in the evening. The ringing stops, and then starts again. It stops and then starts again once more. She's afraid that it is her doctor calling to tell her that he made a mistake and the cancer is back. She gets out of bed and walks slowly toward the phone in the kitchen. She answers tentatively: "Um, hello?" and is surprised to hear Danny's voice. "Mom? What on earth is going on? I've called you about 10 times and you are never there, and you don't return my calls! What is going on? Are you okay?" Mary starts to cry, at first silently and then in loud gulps. Where can she be-gin to tell him how afraid she is, how terrified she is of the future? She's not sure that she even has the words.

It is difficult for some of us to **ask for help**, especially if you have always been the one in your family or social group to whom others have come when they have a problem. Some survivors and their families think that after a certain time, things should be back to normal, and any deviation from this leads to guilt and shame. If you assume that things will be "business as usual" the day after you complete treatment, and two years lat-er you are having difficulties coping physically or emotionally, it may be very difficult to ask for help or seek support. Some cancer survivors feel guilty when they are not coping. They may think they should be grateful for having survived and should not complain about anything. And even worse, sometimes they are told by other people to be happy that treatment is over and grateful that they have survived.

For those who have a **faith-based practice**, attending religious services can be helpful, as this may also serve as a distraction from worry. Placing your faith in a higher power is a common strategy for many people. This can modify the sense of personal responsibility that many cancer survivors place on themselves about recurrence. Participating in church, synagogue, or mosque activities, especially if they involve service to vulnerable communities, can also be helpful because these initiatives take the focus and preoccupation away from you and allow you to give of yourself to others.

> *Mary eventually tells Danny everything. He is shocked at the state she is in and for a moment is speechless. But he is a competent young man, and while he is on the phone, he searches the Internet for the Web site of the cancer center where Mary received her treatment years ago. "Now listen, Mom. They have all sorts of services and programs at the cancer center. They have social workers and groups and things that I think will help you. Can you please call them—I'll give you the number right now—and do something to help yourself?"*
>
> *Mary hesitates. It's been some time since she went to the cancer center, and the doctor said she was finished with them. "I don't know, Danny. I don't go there anymore . . ."*
>
> *Danny is persistent. "I'll tell you what, Mom. If you go and see someone, a social worker maybe, then I'll come down to see you in the next month. Or you can*

come here and stay with Lisa and me. How about that? We haven't seen each other in ages and maybe a break from your routine will do you good."

He can't see it, but she smiles. Her Danny always knew how to creep into her heart. He always knew how to get his way, and the thought of seeing him again, being able to disappear into his hug, is very tempting. Maybe she will make the call, for his sake.

Support groups can be a good way of dealing with fears of recurrence for some people. Different kinds of support groups are available, and it may take a while before you find one that you like and that you find helpful. Support groups may or may not have a formal facilitator. This person may be a professional, such as a social worker, psychologist, or nurse, or may be a layperson who is a cancer survivor. The group may be specific to a kind of cancer, for example, breast cancer, or may be restricted to a certain age group, for example, women younger than 40. Some support groups encourage the participation of family members and friends, whereas others are restricted to only cancer survivors. There are open support groups, where newcomers can join at any time, and closed groups, where membership is restricted to those who joined at a certain time. Some support groups focus on providing information to participants and may have a guest speaker at every meeting with some time allowed for open discussion. Other support groups do not have a formal component and instead allow members to raise issues as they want and then allow the discussion to flow.

All these approaches have pros and cons. A professional acting as a facilitator may keep the content of the meetings strictly controlled, which may not suit those who want to spend more time in general conversation about how they are feeling. Some laypeople can be highly effective facilitators, whereas others may struggle to keep the group on topic or allow their own experiences to color what goes on in the meeting. Some support groups are little more than gripe sessions where participants talk about their negative experiences and the bad things that have happened to them. These kinds of meetings are generally not constructive and may do more harm than good.

Support groups that focus on stress reduction or problem solving have been shown to be more helpful in reducing anxiety than support groups that do not have a specific focus. Before joining a support group, it may be helpful to have a list of questions that can help clarify what happens in the meetings. The answers can help you decide whether this is a group you want to join or if you need to keep looking. Here are some questions that you can ask.

- Does the group have a professional or lay facilitator?
- How long has this person been doing this?
- What is the format of the meetings? Are there guest lecturers or specific topics for each meeting?
- Are family members and friends welcome to attend?
- How much time at each meeting is spent in open discussion?
- What happens when there is conflict between members or a difficult situation arises? Are there mechanisms in place to address this?
- How long do people tend to stay in the group?

Some survivors remain in support groups for many years. Over time, their role in the group may change from that of someone seeking support to someone providing support for newcomers. It is important to reassess your role and what you are getting out of attending a support group every now and then. Going out of habit may not be a good use of your time or energy. You should know when it is time to move on, and you should feel good about that.

There is a risk that going to a support group and hearing about other survivors' experiences may increase your fears. It can also be challenging to witness other survivors' journeys, and a recurrence in someone else may trigger your own fears. If attending a support group makes you feel worse, then you need to either find another group or stop attending. It can be challenging for survivors who live in smaller cities or towns where different options do not exist. A growing number of online support groups exist that meet regularly over the Internet. Members sign on and type in their questions and responses; some even have the capacity for real-time dialogue with microphones and webcams.

Do not worry about hurting the facilitator's or organizer's feelings if you decide not to attend the support group or if you stop going. This is not about their feelings! Your time and energy are valuable, and only you can decide if attending a support group is worth it for you.

TAKE-HOME MESSAGES

What can you learn from this chapter about fear of recurrence? First, it is important to know that being afraid of the cancer coming back is a very common experience and one that does not necessarily go away with time. Fear of recurrence is associated with triggers, internal and external, that may cause intrusive thoughts that can be distressing and negatively affect quality of life.

There are different ways to cope with this fear. Identifying what you are afraid of is an important first step in being able to help yourself cope with the fear. Many strategies are available to help you relax, including refocusing your negative thoughts, progressive muscle relaxation, deep breathing, MBSR, exercise, asking for help from friends and family, finding help in your faith, and attending a support group. You may find that one or a combination of multiple strategies is helpful, no matter how long you have been a survivor. The further away from the time of diagnosis you are, the less your chances of having a recurrence. This is a source of great hope and comfort for many survivors, whereas for others the fear of recurrence never goes away. There is no right or wrong about this; it just is what it is, and you need to find a way to deal with it. Hopefully the suggestions in this chapter will help.

CHAPTER 3

BATTLING THE BLUES

D epression is a fairly common experience in Western society, affecting almost 7% of Americans. Cancer survivors experience depression at a rate that is two to five times greater than the general population, with some studies suggesting that 38% of cancer survivors are depressed. Depression can and does have a negative effect on multiple areas in the lives of people with cancer. It has been suggested that patients with cancer with depression may do worse than nondepressed patients. Increased levels of cancer progression, and ultimately death, among patients with depression have been suggested from a review of more than 9,000 patients with cancer. In another study, patients with depressive symptoms were 25% more likely to die, and those who had been diagnosed by a doctor as having major or minor depression were 40% more likely to die. These are frightening statistics.

WHAT IS DEPRESSION?

Depression is a medical condition with emotional, physical, and behavioral effects. People with depression report feeling sad, losing interest in the things that they previously enjoyed, and feeling worthless. They may have trouble concentrating or making even simple decisions, like what they want to eat for lunch. Some people with depression think about killing or otherwise hurting themselves. Physical manifestations of depression include body aches and pains and lack of energy. Depression can make people act differently. Weight gain or loss due to changes in appetite is common. Some people sleep more when they are depressed, whereas others find that they cannot get to sleep easily and wake often.

Depression is thought to occur in response to a life-changing event such as the loss of a loved one or the diagnosis of a serious illness. This is often called *reactive depression.* Other theories about depression include the belief that depression is caused by an imbalance of chemicals in the brain. Depression covers a wide range of symptoms from the normal sadness experienced in response to loss, to chronic feelings of loss of happiness and joy, and to clinical depression where the feelings and behaviors of the person meet specific criteria.

The following is a list of symptoms that would be used in assessing someone for signs of a major clinical depression. Usually the assessment is made on whether the person has had a depressed mood or loss of pleasure in the same two-week period, in addition to five or more of the following.

- Depressed mood most of the day, nearly every day
- Significant loss of interest or pleasure in all, or almost all, activities most of the day, nearly every day
- Significant weight loss when not dieting or weight gain (such as a change of more than 5% of body weight in a month), or decrease or increase in appetite nearly every day

- Inability to sleep or sleeping excessively nearly every day
- Restlessness (the inability to sit still, pacing, hand-wringing, or pulling or rubbing of the skin, clothing, or other objects) or sluggishness (slowed speech, thinking, and body movements; increased pauses before answering; speech that is decreased in volume, inflection, amount, or variety of content, or muteness) nearly every day
- Fatigue or loss of energy nearly every day
- Feelings of worthlessness or excessive or inappropriate guilt (which may be delusional) nearly every day
- Diminished ability to think or concentrate or difficulty making decisions nearly every day
- Recurrent thoughts of death (not just fear of dying), recurrent thoughts about ending one's life without a specific plan, or a suicide attempt or a specific plan for committing suicide

DEPRESSION AND CANCER

Why does depression happen to cancer survivors when treatment is over? Research tells us that the kind of cancer one has, how bad it was when diagnosed (usually determined by the stage), age at diagnosis (more likely for depression to occur when the person is younger at diagnosis), and whether the person has a strong social and support network can influence the onset of depression early in the disease process. But depression can also happen when treatment is over, a time when most survivors would expect to be, or would be expected by others to be, happy and relieved.

Susan recently completed her 100 days after a stem cell transplant for the treatment of lymphoma and has done well. She has had minimal complications from the transplant, and the doctors have told her they are optimistic about her recovery. The preparation for a stem cell transplant was grueling: first there was the search for a suitable donor, and then she had high doses of chemotherapy to destroy her body's own immune system. She spent many weeks in the hospital and was very sick throughout her stay. Finally, she had the stem cell transplant and waited to see if it was successful. She has now passed the critical 100-day period and is slowly recovering from her long hospital stay. Since coming home, she has spent most of the time inside. She is afraid to go out in case she is exposed to someone who has a cold, the flu, or worse. And she has no energy. She sleeps almost 14 hours at night and falls asleep most afternoons after eating lunch. Her husband, Bill, is baffled: Why is she not getting better? What happened to the Sue who worked full time at the bank, managed their daughter's basketball team, and baked cookies every weekend? He was tired too, and he had really hoped that by now she would be back to her usual routine. Instead she spent most of her time lying on the couch, with the TV on CNN even though she didn't seem to be watching.

As survivors and their families know all too well, the months or even years of treatment are busy ones. There are multiple appointments to see doctors, nurses, and other health professionals. Some people get radiation treatments every day for months in addition to chemotherapy treatments every week for even more months. Any kind of surgery usually requires a hospital stay and at least six weeks of recovery. And then there is the time needed to recover from the treatments and the fatigue from multiple hospital and clinic visits.

And then one day, the treatment phase is over. And the busyness suddenly stops. There may be a lot of empty time in the days and weeks that were once filled with visits to the treatment center. And now there is nothing to fill that empty time. As discussed in Chapter 1, being in treatment can be a comfort in a strange way; the person with cancer is cared for, physically for certain but also often emotionally. Healthcare providers, and the attention they pay to their patients, help to make patients with cancer feel safe in uncertain and scary times. Not seeing those healthcare providers often leaves survivors and their families feeling unsure of what will happen and frightened that they will not know what to do if something goes wrong or if they will even recognize that something is going wrong.

For some, the nurses and other care providers become almost like a second family to the patient. Moving on from treatment means letting go of those relationships, which can be quite intense and meaningful. This can cause sadness and loss for the survivor even though the end of treatment is a good thing. As a survivor, you have to let go of the safety of the treatment center and the intensity of the relationships established there. You also have to start reducing the amount of help-seeking behavior you have been doing over the previous months or years. This is called *de-professionalizing*, cutting the bonds with healthcare professionals, and it can be difficult. You may feel lost and frightened. And you can become depressed and anxious without the safety net of the intensity of care.

Often the pressure from those around you to get back to normal is significant. But what is normal after treatment is over? The chapters of this book describe the many challenges for cancer survivors and point out that life after cancer is not the old normal but rather a new and altered normal for most people. Your spouse or partner may have changed as well. It is not unusual for your spouse or partner to have shouldered extra duties and responsibilities while you were in treatment. For some, this can be empowering with the realization that he or she can take care of the children with the same efficiency and results as you. Or the partner may be surprised to learn that he or she can balance a checkbook and organize your family finances. But often the partner wants to go back to things as they were and is eager to relinquish the extra responsibilities to you as soon as treatment is over. There may be considerable strain too. For the time of treatment, your spouse or partner may have been doing so much that he or she is exhausted and may feel resentful about having to do everything, or what feels like everything. And then the partner feels guilty for thinking and feeling like that, and resentment plus guilt can lead to relationship strain.

> *Sue went for a follow-up appointment to the oncologist. Getting dressed took a major effort. She spent almost 30 minutes deciding what to wear; she just could not make up her mind. On the one hand, she wanted to wear something other than the sweats she had been wearing every day since her discharge from the hospital.*

On the other hand, it seemed like too much work to put on jeans and a sweater. So she sat on her bed, staring into her closet. Eventually she just put on the sweats she had worn all weekend. Her friend Hanna drove her to the appointment and dropped her right outside the clinic doors. She walked slowly toward the elevator, her chest heaving from the effort. One of the nurses who worked with her oncologist joined her at the closed elevator doors. She seemed surprised at how tired Sue looked.

"Are you okay, Sue? Do you need a wheelchair? I can get one quickly."

Sue shook her head. "I'm okay. I just haven't done much since the transplant. It's scary how out of condition I am . . ."

"I'll check in on you when you're done with Dr. Bailey, Sue. Don't leave till you've seen me, okay?"

Some oncologists and nurses routinely assess their patients for signs of depression. They may ask a few questions about mood and daily activity at every visit, or they may use some kind of questionnaire or screening tool that the survivor completes. However, if a healthcare provider doesn't ask how you are coping or feeling, it can be very difficult to bring up the topic yourself. When you are depressed, it can be almost impossible to find the energy to talk about how you are feeling. And so often healthcare providers are very busy, and you don't want to take up too much of their time. You know that there are many people sitting in the waiting room, and you know how hard it is to be one of those people, waiting and waiting. So instead of raising the topic, you let the opportunity to explain how you are feeling or ask for help slip by.

It is also not easy to talk about how you are feeling with your family and friends. Depression is sometimes seen as a weakness, and to admit that you are weak is not easy to do. Many of us have been brought up by parents who lived through tough times, and the message we received growing up was to keep quiet, not complain, and just get on with things. Or we may regard depression as something to be ashamed about, a taboo, and something that should be hidden.

Some people report feeling lonely after the cancer experience. In a study of 13 women treated for breast cancer, a sense of loneliness pervaded their stories of cancer survivorship. They reported that others did not see the significance of the cancer experience in their lives and treated them like heroes or regarded the experience as being over once treatment was over. Being treated as a hero or having a life-altering event dismissed by others made these women feel very alone. In response to this, they did not share their feelings even with those closest to them, such as their sisters or husbands.

How you cope with challenges in life may influence the development of depression. If you naturally have a pessimistic outlook on life, what we often call a "glass-half-empty" outlook, you may be more likely to become depressed when your treatment is over. You may expect the worst to happen, and you interpret how you are feeling more negatively than someone with an optimistic outlook. We often call optimists "glass-half-full" people. They see the bright side of most things and are less likely to suffer from depression when faced with the same challenges as a pessimist. If you use denial as a usual coping mechanism, then depression is also more likely to occur. And if you had problems with depression before your cancer was diagnosed, you are more likely to be depressed both during and after treatment.

> *Sue waited for almost 45 minutes to be called into an exam room. Dr. Bailey seemed hurried—he was running behind—and Sue made sure to only answer the questions he asked her. She didn't say a word about how tired she was and how much she was sleeping. Dr. Bailey spent most of the appointment reviewing the results of her blood tests, and Sue hardly had to say anything. He looked up from her chart, smiled at her, and told her she was doing fine, as well as could be expected—better, actually. And then he was gone.*

Waiting a long time to see your healthcare provider is very common. It's called a waiting room for a good reason! But what tends to happen after all that waiting is that your appointment is rushed and you feel like you do not have the time to ask the questions you need to. So you either ignore them or forget them, and before you know it, the doctor or nurse is out the door and you have to wait until next time.

One thing you can do is write out a list of questions that you have and tell the provider that you have a list of questions you would like to ask. That usually allows the doctor or nurse to make time for your questions in the allotted time of your appointment. You may have to come back again in the near future to address those issues at a separate appointment. Some healthcare providers leave time at the end of the day to see people who need some extra time. But you have every right to have your questions answered to your satisfaction. It is also helpful to have someone with you to write down the answers to your questions. We often don't hear what we are told, especially if we have lots of questions, and a second pair of ears can be very helpful. Some healthcare providers even encourage their patients to record the answers to their questions on tape so that they can review them later.

Sue started to get up after the doctor left the room but then remembered that the nurse—what was her name?—wanted to see her. So she sat down again and waited. About three minutes later, the nurse entered the room.

"Oh, Sue, I'm glad you waited. You seem really tired and I'm worried about that. Can you tell me more about how you are feeling?"

"Um, tired, I guess, really tired. I sleep a lot but I don't seem to be refreshed by my sleep, so I have to nap. Some days it seems that all I do is sleep, and still I feel exhausted. I can tell that Bill is getting tired of me not being back to normal. But I just can't seem to get going."

"Is there anything else, Sue? Are you having bad memories about the transplant or your time in the hospital?"

"Well, I think about it a lot. And I get scared that the transplant will fail and I'll have to do it again. Yes, I remember all of it, and it's so vivid. It upsets me so I try not to think about it, but it's not easy."

> *The nurse, Laurie was her name, took a deep breath:*
> *"Sue, I think you should see our psychologist. It sounds*
> *to me that you are depressed and maybe even have*
> *some elements of something called PTSD."*
>
> *"PTSD? Isn't that what vets get? How could I possi-*
> *bly have PTSD?"*

Post-traumatic stress disorder, or PTSD, is a reaction seen in people who have experienced some kind of traumatic event. We know that many of our combat veterans experience this, and there is a great deal of suffering involved. People who have survived any kind of disaster may experience this, and we now recognize that people who experience a traumatic medical event, such as a heart attack or cancer, can have signs of PTSD too. Commonly, people with PTSD continue to relive the experience. They may have flashbacks to certain aspects of the event in which they recall vividly the sights, sounds, and even smells of the original event. They frequently have problems getting to sleep or staying asleep and have vivid nightmares. People with PTSD are often easily irritated and have a hard time relaxing. They may be hypervigilant—tense, nervous, and jumpy—and may overreact to sudden sounds and movement. Some people with PTSD find it difficult to interact as they used to with friends and family, which can cause tremendous strain in relationships.

For cancer survivors, PTSD may be experienced as flashbacks to all or part of the treatment they had. They may reexperience what it felt like to have chemotherapy or radiation therapy with all the sights, sounds, and smells so that the survivors feel as though they are reliving the treatment over and over. Cancer survivors with signs of PTSD may be very irritable and may fly into a temper at the slightest provocation or even with no provocation at all. They may not sleep well or have nightmares so that they are exhausted during the day. It is important that this be treated, usually with a combination of medication and counseling. If PTSD is left untreated, the individuals may not be able to move on with their lives and ultimately may see their health suffer as a result.

GETTING HELP FOR DEPRESSION

For some, it is not easy asking for or accepting help. But help is available in different forms. You may find that just talking to a nurse or doctor about your feelings may help you. Or perhaps talking to a trusted friend or family member may provide some relief from your feelings of sadness. But you have to be careful about sharing with people who are not professionals and who love and care for you. They may feel powerless to help you, and you may cause them to feel sad or depressed in reaction to your feelings.

Many cancer centers have social workers who are specially educated to support people with cancer, from diagnosis to after treatment. They help and support many survivors and therefore know what can be expected and what suggestions may help you. Some cancer centers also have psychologists and even psychiatrists who are able to prescribe medication.

Sue wasn't sure that she wanted to see a psychologist, or anyone else for that matter. She was shocked that the nurse had suggested there might be some-thing wrong with her head. Didn't all patients with cancer feel tired after their treatments were over? And what was the nurse talking about with PTSD? But in her heart, she knew that something was not right. She could see it in Bill's eyes when he looked at her.

"Okay, I'll see this psychologist. But what is he going to do?"

"Dr. Sinclair is a she," replied Laurie. "She'll ask you some questions and mostly talk to you, I guess. I'm not 100% sure, but some of my patients have been to see her, and they really liked her and said that she helped."

The next day, Sue received a phone call from Dr. Sinclair's office with an appointment date for two weeks later. She almost didn't go when the day came, but Bill had seemed so relieved when she recounted her conversation with the nurse to him. She decided she would give this psychologist one try and that was it.

A number of studies have examined the effectiveness of psychosocial interventions for people with cancer. They all showed that psychoeducational programs providing education and emotional support are effective in treating depression in cancer survivors. The strongest evidence is for something called *cognitive-behavioral therapy,* or CBT. This treatment is defined as any psychological intervention that is relatively brief (weeks or perhaps a few months), focused on specific goals, based on the principles of behavior change, and directed at making changes in a specific area of concern to the patient. One of the strengths of CBT is that it teaches the survivors to solve their problems and also challenges rigid thinking that often spirals out of control. By reframing negative thoughts and attitudes, people learn to change their negative thought patterns and also their actions. CBT is often called *talk therapy*, but its focus on reframing the negative and altering behavior makes it different from the "lie down on the couch and tell me your earliest memories" kind of talk therapy that is practiced by psychoanalysts.

For Sue, CBT may focus on improving her sleep (the goal) by identifying what is making her so tired and what she is gaining by sleeping for so many hours. It may be that sleep allows her to avoid thinking about her cancer and the treatment. The process of preparing for and recovering from a stem cell transplant is challenging; most people find coping with the chemotherapy to be very difficult, and the extended hospital stay associated with the transplant can be isolating, lonely, and frightening. Identifying the reason *why* she needs to sleep so much and if in fact she is using sleep as a coping or escape mechanism will help Sue to address underlying feelings and more effective methods to cope with what has happened to her (behavior change in a specific area of the person's life).

Psychotherapy and counseling are other interventions that can be helpful to cancer survivors. These differ from CBT in that the focus is more on verbal interactions between the survivor and the therapist or counselor than on reframing and behavior change. These may occur as a result of deeper understanding on the part of the survivor, but they are not the goal of the therapy. *Crisis intervention* is an example of a psychotherapy technique in which the counselor helps the survivor deal with a crisis. The recurrence of cancer may cause the survivor to go into crisis mode, and a skilled therapist would help the person to cope with this change through supportive exchanges.

Information and education are other interventions that can be helpful in alleviating depression, especially if a lack of understanding on the part of the cancer survivor is contributing to the depression. Depression can result from not knowing the facts about the cancer and thinking the worst based on that lack of knowledge. Cancer survivors who are fully informed experience less depression and anxiety than those who are not well informed. Much of the information that cancer survivors receive from their healthcare team is given at the time of diagnosis or when treatment starts. We know that after hearing the words "you have cancer," most people are only able to absorb about 10% of what they are told next. Ten percent! And there is so much information that patients have to somehow read, learn, and understand.

Healthcare providers try to be efficient in giving this information and education, but they are often not aware of where the patient's concentration is focused at the time. So they talk and talk, perhaps even draw a picture or diagram, and then they think that their job is done and that they have told you what you need to know. And so they don't ask if you understood or remember or have questions. Some people spend hours and days and weeks learning more about their cancer and its treatments from a variety of sources. The Internet can provide an abundance of information, but not all of it is valid or accurate. Some people ask other patients for information, or they ask friends or relatives who have had cancer, often a different kind of cancer, about their experience. What you learn from these sources can be comforting and inspiring, but it can also be frightening and not applicable to your situation. Everyone's cancer is different, and everyone's response to treatment is different.

When treatment is over, it may be a good idea to sit down with your doctor or nurse and go over the details of your cancer and treatment. In Chapter 6 you will read about the value of a survivorship care plan. An important part of that care plan is information about the type of cancer and the details of the treatment you had. The care plan also should identify the possible effects of those treatments, both short and long term. Knowing this information can help you to have a realistic understanding of your disease and what could happen. This education and information can help to dispel any misunderstanding or myths you may have heard and may help to address one of the root causes of your depression.

> *Sue went to the appointment with the psychologist. Dr. Sinclair asked her a lot of questions and then suggested that she try some medication to help her sleep better. She said that Sue was probably not getting good quality sleep, and she thought a mild antidepressant could help. Sue wasn't sure this was what she wanted; she was tired of taking pills and wanted to feel like a person and not a patient. When Dr. Sinclair explained that she would ask Sue's own doctor to write the prescription for the medication, Sue decided that she didn't want to do this, and she left the psychologist's office.*

Medications can help in treating depression, and a variety of antidepressants are available. Research shows that antidepres-

sants can be helpful to cancer survivors, and many survivors benefit from them. There is no research to suggest that one medication is better than the other. The physician determines which
antidepressant to use based on the particular drug's side effect
profile. Tricyclic antidepressants, an older class of antidepressants, have a sedating effect and so are helpful to people who are
having difficulties with sleep. A newer class of antidepressants is
the selective serotonin reuptake inhibitors, and these tend to
have fewer side effects, although they are not side effect free.
Some of these medications also help to reduce anxiety, which
can be helpful to some survivors. It can take three to four weeks
to notice any difference in mood, and many people get frustrated waiting to see if the medication is helping. Many survivors
need to have the dose of the medication adjusted so that they
get the maximum benefit with the fewest side effects, and this
can take some time to figure out.

> Later that week, Laurie, the nurse, called Sue to see
> how the appointment with the psychologist had gone.
> She sounded surprised that Sue had not wanted to take
> any medication, and there was a long pause in the call.
> "Um, okay, so do you think you're depressed? Do
> you want to do something about it?" Laurie asked.
> "I don't know if I'm depressed. You're the experts
> here and you seem to think that I am! All I know is that
> I am tired all the time and that I need to sleep."
> "But sleeping doesn't seem to be working for you,"
> replied Laurie. "And the need to sleep may be a sign
> that you are depressed. I'm really not trying to push
> medication on you, but I see someone who is not re-

covering as you should. Would you consider another kind of intervention that might help?"

"Like what?" Sue responded. "I don't mean to be difficult, but I'm tired and I don't have much patience. The psychologist just wanted to give me pills, and I really want my body to just be left alone. If there's something that doesn't involve medication or talking, then maybe I'll try. But I'm too tired to talk."

Some other interventions are available that may be helpful in alleviating depression in cancer survivors, but we don't have strong evidence to support them. One intervention that does seem to help reduce both depression and anxiety in cancer survivors is exercise. This may sound counterintuitive—when you feel down, the last thing you want to do is get up and exercise—but evidence has shown that exercise has all sorts of benefits. First, exercise releases chemicals in the brain that elevate mood. Exercise also lowers chemicals in the immune system that make depression worse, and it raises your body temperature, which seems to have a calming effect. Exercise can be a distraction from the worry that often accompanies depression and is a healthy coping mechanism rather than a negative one, like overeating or avoidance.

And you don't even have to break much of a sweat to see the benefits. Any kind of exercise counts: walking, lifting weights, washing the car, gardening, biking around the neighborhood, or yoga—anything that gets you moving will show results. You may also find that once you start, it is hard to stop, and you want to exercise more and more. You don't even have to do all your exercise in one time period; you can break up the goal of

30 minutes a day into three 10-minute exercise sessions. And doing different kinds of exercise helps to prevent boredom, which in turn increases motivation and sticking to it.

Some people prefer to exercise alone, whereas others find that exercising with a friend or family member keeps them on track with the added benefit of having company. It's easy to talk yourself out of going but is harder to persuade a friend not to go and get it done.

Some other activities, often referred to as *complementary therapies*, have shown benefits for cancer survivors. Massage therapy has been shown to reduce anxiety in cancer survivors, and depressive symptoms were reduced by 50% 2–24 hours after a massage in one study. A small study has also found relaxation training in the form of progressive muscle relaxation (described in Chapter 2) to reduce anxiety and depression. Guided imagery as part of the relaxation also may be helpful.

> *Sue decided that she would give the massage therapy a try. The thought of exercise really didn't appeal to her, and even though her doctor had told her that her risk of getting an infection from crowds was minimal, she didn't want to do anything that involved going out or being with people. She made an appointment with her sister's massage therapist. She had never had a massage in her life, and she was a little embarrassed about taking off her clothes in front of a stranger. But the massage therapist put her at ease on the phone and suggested that she wear a bathing suit if she wanted. Sue almost laughed out loud, but it helped put her at ease, and she found herself looking forward to this new experience.*

TAKE-HOME MESSAGES

Depression is a common side effect of cancer and its treatments; some studies say that more than one-third of cancer survivors experience depression. This can cause great emotional pain and suffering, not only for the survivors but also for the family and friends who love them. And depression has been linked to poorer outcomes for survivors who suffer from it. Treatment of depression is available and includes a variety of talk therapies including CBT, psychotherapy, and information sharing and education. Some survivors, especially those with major depression, will benefit from taking antidepressants, which are highly effective in treating both depression and anxiety. Other strategies may help too. Exercise has been shown to lift mood, among other benefits (see Chapter 5). Massage therapy and progressive relaxation are also beneficial in managing depression. All of these interventions have research to support them, and they are all readily available should you need them. The most difficult part may be asking for help.

CHAPTER 4

WALKING THROUGH MUD

C ancer-related fatigue is a problem for 99% of people with cancer. It starts during treatment of any kind but is worse with chemotherapy and radiation therapy than surgery. It often persists for many months or even years after treatment is over. In one study, 33% of cancer survivors reported a two-week period of fatigue in the previous month more than five years after completing treatment. The reason why fatigue persists long after treatment is over is more difficult to understand than the reasons for fatigue during treatment. But the outcome for cancer survivors is that they are often very tired at a time when they expect and want to feel better.

Cancer-related fatigue is different from any other kind of fatigue because it is not helped by rest or sleep and is greater in magnitude and persists longer than would be expected with fatigue for any other reason, such as exercise-induced fatigue. It also affects survivors' ability to participate in activities that promote health, like exercise, and makes it very difficult for them to adhere to programs that help in long-term recovery. It is widely accepted by experts that potentially many different reasons exist for this fatigue, including both psychological and physical mechanisms. The type of treatment, the stage of disease at diagnosis, and sleep disturbances during and following treatment also can affect how bad the fatigue is and how long it lasts after treatment is over.

WHAT DOES THIS FATIGUE FEEL LIKE?

Cancer survivors who experience this fatigue will tell you that it feels like no other kind they have ever experienced. One survivor described it as "walking through mud"; the fatigue felt like it came from the very depths of her being and was present all day, every day and affected every aspect of her life. Survivors who are fatigued find it difficult to complete daily tasks such as cooking or bathing/showering. They may feel too tired to eat, which can negatively affect nutritional status and further exacerbate energy levels. Return to work may be impossible. This in turn will have an impact on financial security and feelings of competence and usefulness within the family. Survivors may experience changes to their usual sleep patterns with either insomnia (difficulty falling or staying asleep) or sleeping excessive amounts and not feeling restored or refreshed upon waking. They may find it very difficult to do anything other than sit or lie down. This inertia is difficult to deal with, and family and friends may find it confusing or frustrating. This fatigue often causes difficulties with mental activity such as concentration or decision making and is associated with problems with short-term memory. Some survivors also report that their limbs feel weak or heavy. People often experience a significant emotional response to the feelings of fatigue, including frustration and irritability.

Some cancer survivors do not mention their fatigue to their healthcare providers, assuming it is part of what life after cancer holds. And healthcare providers may not ask survivors whether they are fatigued or what their energy levels are like, so a crucial trigger for intervention is missed. This is an important symptom for survivors to discuss with their healthcare provider, especially because things can be done to improve the situation, which will be discussed later in this chapter.

Jim is 48 years old and was treated with surgery, radiation, and chemotherapy for colon cancer. He had a colostomy for a while and was really happy when he had another surgery to reverse that, and now he no longer has to worry about having a bag on his abdomen. What Jim didn't expect was that it would take him so long to recover from the treatment. Four months after the final surgery, he is still exhausted almost every waking moment of the day, and he can't remember the last time he felt like doing anything or going anywhere. He had hoped to be back at work as a high school teacher by now, but he can't imagine being able to stand in front of the class for more than six hours a day. In fact, most days he doesn't get out of bed until well after his wife has left for her job and even after their teenagers have rolled out of bed. He feels guilty about this and wants to help around the house, but even showering in the morning takes all his energy, and he finds himself lying down on the unmade bed wrapped in a bath towel. He hopes that Marilyn, his wife, doesn't catch him resting after his shower; he's sure that she would not be pleased.

WHAT PLAYS A ROLE IN THIS FATIGUE?

Many factors play a role in fatigue in cancer survivors. Depression is a well-known contributor to the experience of fatigue, and, in turn, being fatigued can play a role in depression. As discussed in the previous chapter, fatigue is one of the signs of depression and contributes to feeling depressed as well. The two are interconnected, and their symptoms may mimic each other. However, some very real differences are important to note. First, fatigue itself is not associated with feelings of low self-worth or impending doom or feeling empty and dead inside; these are symptoms of depression and should not be ignored. People who are depressed and receive effective treatment for their depression may remain fatigued despite improvements in their mood and outlook.

If symptoms such as pain and shortness of breath persist after treatment is over, these commonly affect the persistence of fatigue. Some specific treatment-related causes of fatigue also may continue into the post-treatment period. These include anemia, or reduced levels of red blood cells, as a result of chemotherapy or poor nutrition. Red blood cells carry oxygen around the body. Symptoms of anemia include decreased exercise tolerance and endurance, as well as shortness of breath in addition to feeling tired. Levels of red blood cells usually return to normal after treatment is over. The levels of these cells are usually checked when you have blood tests as part of follow-up care, so this cause of fatigue is usually identified as part of routine care. Your immune system also may play a role in the development of fatigue. Cytokines are cells that play a role in controlling inflammation. These can be affected by cancer treatment or the cancer itself, leading to an excess of cytokines, which has been implicated in the development of both fatigue and depression. High levels of cytokines are known to affect not only energy levels but also sleep, cognition, and interest in pleasurable aspects of life, including sex, and may lead to social isolation. These are all affected in someone who is depressed. Much is still to be learned about these complex mechanisms. Research is ongoing in an attempt to understand how the immune system affects fatigue and vice versa.

Related to this is the issue of significant weight loss that may have occurred during chemotherapy or advanced disease. Once again, cytokines are involved in muscle wasting and loss of body fat. People who lose a lot of weight during treatment are known to experience severe fatigue as a result of the increased effort required to use the muscles of the body to achieve any action, such as those used in activities of daily living.

You may have some ongoing issues with pain as a result of the cancer or treatment. Some treatments cause joint pain and stiffness, which can affect your mood and ability to engage in life and lifestyle changes to improve quality of life. You should not suffer in silence, nor should you worry about issues of addiction to pain killers. Being in pain and immobile is worse for you than taking medication. Chronic pain is debilitating and a cause of fatigue and exhaustion, as well as depression and anxiety.

Jim has tried to figure out why he's so tired. He knows that he has been to hell and back during treat-

ment; the surgery was bad, he had to deal with the colostomy, and the radiation was no walk in the park. And then the chemo took whatever was left. He is much thinner than he used to be, and he can see in the mirror that he's lost a lot of muscle mass in his upper body. He still has no appetite and has to force himself to eat while no one is around. Marilyn makes sure he eats dinner, but when she's at work, a bowl of cereal is about all he can manage, and he hardly ever finishes it. He wants to help around the house so badly; he's not bringing in any money, and they have started taking money out of the savings account for household expenses. He feels guilty about this, but what can he do? If he can't even put in a load of laundry, how can he go back to work? Marilyn has asked him a couple of times if he's depressed, but he really doesn't think he is. But he does not feel like himself, that's for sure.

Every day Jim hopes that he will feel better, and every day it's the same. He has no energy and can barely stay awake after dinner. He regularly dozes off in front of the TV. It's become a bit of a family joke, especially when he fell asleep during the Super Bowl game. The kids were shocked; they were yelling and celebrating when their team scored a touchdown, and their dad was snoring gently in his chair.

Marilyn has tried to make suggestions to help him, but nothing seems to help. Now they don't talk about it, as it just causes conflict. She wants him to try to do more, and he can't find the energy or even interest. When she does encourage him to get out more, he just looks at her with his brown eyes that seem even larger now that his face is so thin. He shaves just two or three times a week, so his cheeks are shadowed by his beard and his face looks even thinner. Soon after his surgery, she invited their friends Paul and Maddie for dinner, and Jim almost fell asleep at the table. He hardly contributed to the talk around the table, and there were awkward silences where once he would have been telling jokes and teasing their guests. She is at her wit's end, and he doesn't seem to notice or care.

WHAT CAN BE DONE ABOUT IT?

Experts have looked at a number of different interventions to help survivors get over this fatigue. Some interventions have been helpful, while others have shown little or no benefit. First, it is important to tell your healthcare provider about any fatigue you are experiencing. They need to assess what might be causing it, for example, anemia, and treat that as part of the plan to get you back on track in your recovery. If you are depressed, treating the depression with cognitive-behavioral therapy and/or medication is an important step. Alleviating the depression may be what you need to find the motivation to get off the couch or out of bed and into an exercise program. A useful tool for describing your level of fatigue is the following scale.

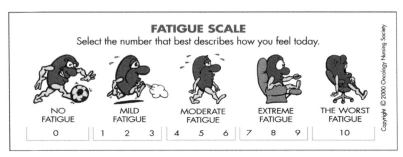

Note. Copyright 2000 by the Oncology Nursing Society. Used with permission.

As you can see, the scale goes from 0 (no fatigue) to 10 (the worst fatigue) and can help you track improvements in your fatigue. Feel free to make a copy of this and carry it with you or place it with your exercise log (more about that in Chapter 5).

> *At his last appointment with the surgeon, Jim admitted that it was taking longer than expected to feel like his old self. The doctor stopped examining him and asked:*
>
> *"Is there something bothering you, Jim? You certainly haven't gained any weight back and you don't seem like yourself, even the self I knew when you first came to see me. I think maybe you should talk to your primary care provider. Or there's this new rehab program at the hospital where you had your surgery. Maybe that would help. By now you should be back at work . . ."*
>
> *"How would rehab help? I can barely stay awake after my morning shower."*
>
> *"That's the point, Jim. We understand that after cancer, some patients need an active program of rehabil-*

itation to get them back on their feet. Why don't you give it a try?"

Jim sighed. He knew in his heart that he needed to do something; he just couldn't figure out what that something was supposed to be. He supposed he could look into it. But that was all he could do for now.

It is always helpful for survivors to learn how to manage their fatigue, and this includes involving your family and friends in educational sessions or reading educational material about fatigue and its management.

A first step that can be helpful is learning how to **conserve energy and actively manage the fatigue**. It is important to balance rest and activity, and some people need more help in doing this than others. Survivors may push themselves too hard in an attempt to get back to normal and, in doing so, may be making the fatigue worse, or at least not helping.

You may need to enlist the help and support of your family to remind you when you need to rest and motivate you to be active—but then you have to listen to them and not make them feel bad for trying to help! Sometimes, family just can't be firm enough to push you in the right direction. They may be too concerned to help you do what you need to do and love you too much to be firm with you when you need it most. And they are survivors too and may also be tired, both physically and emotionally, from the months or years of supporting you through treatment.

Here are some suggestions to help you conserve energy.

- Decide what is important to you and then prioritize. Is taking a shower more important than dusting? Remember, someone else can do the dusting, but only you can shower your-self!

- Ask for help, even though it is hard to do. Asking family members or friends to do a specific task can be helpful to them as well as you. They want to help, and being told what to do often makes them feel helpful.

- Pace yourself and take frequent breaks. Ten minutes of sorting out bills and paperwork can be rewarded with a five-minute break for a glass of juice or a granola bar.

- Plan what you want to achieve and be realistic. You are not going to be able to clear the backlog of mail sitting in piles on your desk in one session. Perhaps you can start with discarding the junk mail for just 20 minutes. Then the next day you can deal with a cleaner desk with fewer piles and another goal, perhaps this time organizing get-well cards that need to be answered.

- Sit and stand with good posture. Slumping or hunching may cause muscular and joint problems. Make sure that you do some gentle stretches when you take a break, and remember to breathe with your abdominal muscles.

- Avoid extremes in temperature, such as cold or hot outdoors and overheated or cooled interiors. Be especially careful about moving from one to the other frequently.

- Some people find that massage therapy, healing touch, and relaxation exercises help to restore energy, although studies have not shown these to have a significant or lasting effect.

Jim took the pamphlet about the rehab program that the doctor gave him. He wasn't sure that he was all that interested, but when Marilyn saw it, she became excited.

"This sounds wonderful, honey! Are you going to go?"

"Um, I don't know. I haven't really thought about it, and I don't really have the energy to talk about it now. I need to have a nap."

Marilyn took a deep breath, opened her mouth, and then closed it again. She was tired too, and she didn't have the energy to push him anymore. He always did exactly what he wanted anyway, and it was useless to fight with him. But she knew she had to do something. She decided she would call this rehab program to learn more about it and perhaps even find out if there was anything she could do to help him.

She called the number listed on the pamphlet the next day during her mid-morning break. The person who answered the phone identified himself as Mark and said that he was an exercise specialist. She was not sure what that meant, maybe a fancy name for a personal trainer, but he sounded nice. He encouraged her to come to an information session they were having at the rehab center later that week. She told Jim that she was going about an hour before she left the house, and for an instant she thought that maybe he would come with her, but her hopes were dashed when he just shrugged and told her to "have fun."

She learned a lot that evening. Mark, the exercise specialist, led the meeting, and as his voice suggested, he was friendly and warm. Most of the people there were in couples, and she felt out of place being alone. But she was soon drawn into what was being said and forgot that she had no one with her. Everything she had thought about Jim's recovery was wrong, completely wrong! What he needed wasn't more rest; he needed to get moving. It sounded weird, but Mark was really convincing. Now how was she going to get Jim to go along with what seemed like his best chance to get better?

The most effective strategy to combat cancer-related fatigue is **exercise**. Many people would find that surprising: how can someone who is totally exhausted find the energy to exercise? It almost sounds counterintuitive; when you're tired, you need to rest, not do something that makes you even more tired! But exercise has been shown to be highly effective in reducing cancer-related fatigue in a number of studies. The experts agree that some combination of aerobic activity (think walking or gardening) and resistance training (light weights or elastic bands) is optimal for a post-treatment exercise regimen. The topic of exercise (and nutrition) will be explored in great detail in Chapter 5, but here are some general principles about how and when to incorporate exercise into your life as a way of relieving fatigue.

Exercise can help treat depression and improve mood. It also improves muscle strength, which in turn reduces muscle fatigue and the effort needed to do everyday tasks and activities. Exercise helps you sleep better and keeps your weight under control. All of this will help combat fatigue.

As with all behavior changes, think about rewarding yourself at key points as you make changes. The reward doesn't have to cost a lot of money and, in fact, may not cost anything at all. But set some goals for yourself and do something when you reach them. Reward is a strong motivator. You deserve it!

Many cancer survivors make significant changes to their **diet** when they are diagnosed. Carrying these into survivorship can add not only years to your life by preventing the diseases associated with obesity and unhealthy food choices, but they may actually improve the quality of your life and give you energy and a feeling of general wellness. Details about how nutrition plays a role in survivorship will be provided in Chapter 5, but remember that food is the fuel that allows your body to function, heal, and do what it needs to do.

Marilyn's efforts to encourage Jim seemed to be paying off. After the meeting at the rehab center, she repeated exactly what Mark had said. She saw something that looked like a spark of interest in Jim's eyes when she explained how even though it sounded strange, just doing something to get moving could— no, would—help in the long run. Jim had been the quarterback for his high school and college football teams, and he had a very competitive spirit. She was not sure what she had said, but the next day he went for a walk after dinner. It was only around the block and he was gone for close to 20 minutes, but there was something in his eyes when he came back. The next evening he went again, and this time she offered to go with him even though she had a ton of laundry to do. And before either of them knew it, their after-dinner walk had become a regular thing. The night before they had even held hands as they walked and talked, and she realized that they were really talking as they walked, not just making comments in passing about the kids or her work. This felt good!

Jim had noticed a change too. He was sleeping better since they started the nightly walks. They were walking farther, too, and his pace had quickened enough that Marilyn was taking longer strides to keep up. He didn't wake up nearly so often in the night, and he was able to shower and dress without having to rest. Even his appetite had improved; he actually thought about what he would have for lunch, where before the thought of eating didn't cross his mind. Maybe, after all this time, he had turned a corner, and he didn't mean just the corner at the end of the block.

Another very important factor in fatigue is **sleep**, both in quality and quantity. Poor quality sleep is a major contributor to fatigue, whereas good quality sleep can help you feel rested and energized. When survivors are sleeping poorly, they often try to compensate by taking one or more naps during the day or are so exhausted that they fall asleep even though they do not plan to. Long naps and naps later in the day affect sleep quality at night, as well as delay the onset of sleepiness at night time. Here are some suggestions for establishing good habits for sleep.

- Avoid naps longer than 20 minutes.
- Do not nap late in the afternoon or early in the evening.
- Try to set a consistent time for going to bed and for getting up.

- Establish a pre-bed routine, such as having a warm shower or bath or reading for 15 minutes, and do this consistently.
- Do not watch TV in bed; the bedroom is for sleep and sex only.
- Avoid caffeine, sodas, and alcohol in the evenings, as these are stimulants.
- If you wake in the middle of the night, go to another room and read in dim lighting until you feel sleepy. Don't turn on the TV or use the computer because this will stimulate your brain.

It can take some time to get this right. Be patient and try not to get stressed about not sleeping, even though it can be stressful. Taking sleep medication may be a temporary solution if your sleep is very poor. However, like all medications, sleeping pills can have side effects and can be both physically and mentally addictive. A number of natural remedies and herbal treatments claim to promote sleep, but most have not been studied extensively. Just because they are "natural" does not mean that they don't have side effects.

There has been some research into the usefulness of **medication** to treat cancer-related fatigue. These medications include stimulants and antidepressants. They do have significant side effects, however, and are not widely used in the absence of good studies supporting their use.

An interesting study on the use of **mindfulness-based cognitive therapy** has shown good results in treating fatigue. The mindfulness program consisted of nine weeks of sessions where mindfulness techniques were taught and then practiced at home for 45 minutes a day, six days a week. The program combined sitting and walking exercises as described in Chapter 5. Participants in the study who attended the sessions and did the homework reported improved fatigue, greater well-being, and less impairment of their functional abilities, and the effects lasted for at least six months. The program and homework were time intensive and may not be appropriate or possible for everyone.

Jim made great strides in his recovery once he started sleeping and eating better. Every day his fatigue seemed to be less of a problem, and he had more energy to do things around the house. He even made an appointment to see his primary care provider to be cleared to go back to work. He called the principal, who seemed really happy to hear from him. Wally was an old friend from college, and although they had chosen different paths in the teaching world (Jim loved the classroom and Wally couldn't wait to get into school administration), they had a long history.

"Any time you're ready, buddy. I can tell you we're ready to have you back. The kids have missed you too, and they've been giving some of the substitutes a hard time . . . but you don't need to hear that! Just come back anytime."

Jim did need to hear that. It felt good to know that "his" kids missed him. As he put the phone down, he looked at the calendar on the office wall. Next week was the spring break, and maybe he could go back after that. He couldn't wait for Marilyn to come home so that he could talk to her as they walked that evening. He was looking forward to seeing her face when he told her.

TAKE-HOME MESSAGES

Fatigue is a common and debilitating consequence of cancer and its treatment. It affects all aspects of daily life and can delay healing and recovery. The most effective and proven treatment for cancer-related fatigue is exercise. This chapter has described the principles of exercise as a strategy to combat fatigue, and greater detail will be provided in the next chapter, along with information about nutrition. Getting a good night's sleep regularly can also help; however, sleep problems often go hand in hand with fatigue. Other strategies to help with fatigue are identifying and treating the cause of fatigue, such as anemia or depression. Massage therapy, relaxation exercises, and mindfulness-based therapy have also been shown to be helpful. However, the use of medication is not recommended. The next chapter will cover exercise and diet in more detail.

CHAPTER 5

MOVING RIGHT ALONG

M any people who are diagnosed with cancer make significant changes to their lives, and sometimes their family members do, too. Cancer can be a very real wake-up call for many, and with the diagnosis comes the impetus to take better care of oneself. Many of those affected by cancer seek ways to improve their diet, sometimes looking for something to control when everything else seems uncontrollable. This chapter will present the latest information on lifestyle factors that are important to cancer survivors. Exercise, nutrition, smoking cessation, moderation in alcohol consumption, and sun protection are lifestyle factors that cancer survivors and their families need to pay attention to, but care must be taken to get it right.

WHAT ABOUT NUTRITION?

There is no magic diet or food that will cure cancer. Despite the promises of miracles in countless ads (usually in the back of magazines), nothing you eat or avoid eating will cure cancer. It is as simple as that, even though some people would like to think otherwise. But a balanced and high-quality diet can help you stay healthy, prevent obesity, and, for the cancer survivor, help the body to repair itself and heal after treatment. A healthy, balanced diet will also help you feel better, fight infection, and help you to regain your strength and get back to the new normal of life after cancer.

Increasing evidence shows that obesity is linked to cancer, although what that link is seems to be less clear. We know that when a person with cancer is obese, the prognosis is poorer than if the person were of healthy weight. It stands to reason that cancer survivors need to maintain a healthy weight, both in terms of the cancer but also for heart health and the myriad other reasons why obesity poses a very significant risk to health and well-being. Obesity is linked to heart disease and diabetes, two conditions that kill millions of people in North America every year, and surviving cancer does *not* mean that you are immune to other threats to your health and life.

> *Barry is a hard-working, hard-playing stockbroker who, at the age of 53, was diagnosed with esophageal cancer. The diagnosis came as a shock, and his treatment journey was complicated by his anger at his body letting him down. Barry would be considered by anyone who met him as a classic type A personality; he is brash and confident and has a short temper and even less patience with himself and others. He struggled with having to have radiation and chemotherapy and refused to talk to anyone, including his wife, Elaine, about how he was feeling. He was unable to eat for most of the six weeks of radiation and lost almost 45 pounds.*

Now that his treatment is over, he has no energy and no stamina. He went to work every day during his treatment even though he was not very productive most of the time. Now that his treatment is over, he is frustrated that he is not back to making his usual 120% effort. Elaine has tried to help him in every way she can imagine, and now her efforts are focused on helping him gain back the weight he lost.

The key to a **balanced diet** is to eat a variety of foods with a focus on plant-based foods such as colorful fruits and vegetables, which contain the most nutrients. These should be the mainstay of your diet, with other food groups in smaller quantities. When you are at the market, zone in on the fruits and vegetables that glow with deep, rich color: deep green kale and spinach (forget about that wintry white iceberg lettuce in its plastic cover!). Buy lots of orange and red fruits and vegetables: apples, red peppers, and oranges; the darker the color, the higher the nutritional value. You should eat 8–10 servings of fruit and vegetables a day, which sounds like a lot, but one serving is only half a cup. So you need to eat four to five cups a day of these nutritious and tasty fresh items. Remember that it is always better to eat fruits and vegetables in their whole form rather than in juice. The juice does not contain any fiber, and many packaged fruit juices contain added sugar that just adds calories and no nutritional value.

Whole grains and legumes (beans, etc.) should be the next group by quantity. You need to read the labels carefully and look for food that has the words "whole grains" in the first two ingredients. Just because something is brown does not mean it is whole grain. White flour can be made to look like brown flour, but that does not mean it contains whole grains. It is recommended that you eat at least three servings of whole grains a day, which is easier than you think. One serving of whole grains is a single slice of whole grain bread (look for bread that has seeds and nuts clearly visible in the slices), so a sandwich for lunch would give you two servings. Half a cup of whole grain pasta or brown rice is a serving, and a whole grain pita or bagel gives you two servings. See how quickly they add up? Think about adding legumes to your diet, too. Black-eyed peas, navy beans, and soy beans are examples of legumes. Beans and lentils are powerhouses of nutrition that add fiber to your diet along with a good source of complex carbohydrates that supply energy over the day.

Protein is important to the body because it helps with healing and rebuilding muscle, something that might have been lost during treatment, especially if you have lost a lot of weight. But you need much less protein than you may think: just one cup per day. That's about the size of a pack of playing cards. Try to eat lean protein (fish and the white meat of chicken without the skin), and limit your intake of red meat (beef, lamb, and pork) to two servings a week. Dairy products count as proteins. These should be limited to low-fat or nonfat products. Watch how much cheese you eat—a portion is the size of two dice—because cheese contains a lot of fat.

As a cancer survivor, you need to limit how much fat you eat, especially the saturated fat that is found in meats and cheeses. Any fat that is solid at room temperature is a saturated fat, like butter, cheese, and lard. You need to keep your fat intake to below 50 grams per day. Fat is often hidden in prepared

foods. Be careful about prepared salad dressings, commercial-
ly prepared baked goods, and margarine; they contain high
amounts of saturated fats and salt. Monounsaturated fats, however, are much better for you. Any fat that is liquid at room
temperature is usually monounsaturated, such as olive oil and
canola oil. Avocadoes and nuts are good sources of these kinds
of fats, but remember that they are still fats and must be count-
ed in your daily intake of less than 50 grams.

You need to be a savvy **label reader**. Almost all foods today
(except fresh fruits and vegetables and raw meat) have a label, which can be a useful tool in making smart food choices. First, look at the serving size. You may be surprised that
the suggested serving size is much smaller than what you
would normally eat. A bag of cookies may list a serving size
as one cookie, and you usually eat five or six at a time! Then
look at how many calories are listed per serving, and multi-
ply that by how many servings you intend to eat. The label
also will tell you what percentage of your daily requirements
is in each serving; this is based on a 2,000-calorie diet. The
amount of fat per serving will be given as a total and then as
the amount of saturated and unsaturated fats. Try to eat only
foods that have low saturated fat and avoid trans-fats completely; these are known to be very bad for our bodies and are
now banned in many products. Try to eat foods that are high
in fiber (check the fiber count as well as the percentage of fiber per serving). Next, look at the list of ingredients. Those
listed first are found in the biggest proportion in that item.
If sugar (glucose, fructose, sucrose, corn syrup) is in the first
three listed ingredients, step away from the package! Be very
careful about foods that are advertised as "low fat." They of-

ten contain high amounts of sugar and may not be that different from the regular version of the food, but the serving size may be much smaller than in the regular product.

How you **cook** your food is also important. Try to steam, poach, bake, or boil your food instead of frying. Be careful about grilling meat because when protein burns (those crispy bits on the edges of a steak), it turns into chemicals that have been linked to the development of cancer. If your meat is burned, cut off those pieces and do not eat the charred bits (even though they are tasty). As a cancer survivor, you also need to limit your intake of smoked and pickled foods. These contain high levels of nitrates, which are linked to cancer.

There has been a lot of talk about **super foods**, nutrient-rich foods that are supposed to play a role in cancer prevention. Nutrient-rich foods may help you to get and stay healthy, but no evidence has shown that they play a role in the prevention of cancer or its recurrence. Nutrient-rich foods contain vitamins, minerals, antioxidants, and phytochemicals, which are all good for your health. They include colorful fruits and vegetables, citrus fruits such as oranges and grapefruit, cruciferous vegetables such as broccoli and kale, berries, and Brazil nuts. Wild salmon (rather than farmed), sardines, black cod, and striped bass can be eaten two to three times a week. Flaxseed and other legumes are also included because of the fiber they provide. Yogurt with natural cultures (once again, check the label) is thought to keep the immune system healthy. Black, green, and white teas are better for you than soda or caffeinated drinks.

People often wonder if they need to eat only **organic food**. No evidence has demonstrated that organic food is better or more nutritious than regular food. But organic food is produced and processed very differently. For food to be certified as organic, the farmer has to prove that he or she is not using pesticides on fruits and vegetables and that animals for slaughter have not been given antibiotics or growth hormones; these are usual practices for nonorganic farmers. Many people think that the produce available at farmers' markets is organic, but this is not so. You should check with the individual farmers at these markets about their use of pesticides and herbicides. Organic foods are usually more expensive than regular foods in the supermarket and tend to spoil quicker, so you should buy small quantities more often to ensure freshness and minimize waste. They also may not be available in smaller cities and towns, although they are increasingly becoming more popular.

Visiting a farmers' market can expose you to different varieties of fruits and vegetables than you usually see in your supermarket. Fruits and vegetables that have been grown close to where they are sold usually are fresher than those that have been airfreighted and trucked from many miles away or another country. It's also fun to talk to the farmers and their families who bring their produce to the market, and you will learn about different kinds of produce, which may tempt you to try something different. Produce from the farmers' market usually is less clean than what you buy in the supermarket, so make sure to wash and dry it well to get rid of any dirt or tiny critters that have made the journey from the field to your kitchen.

The U.S. Department of Agriculture recommends the following as a guideline for healthy eating (see www.choosemyplate.gov). The Web site contains a wealth of information and resources to help you eat better.

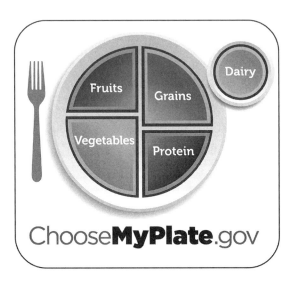

1. Balancing Calories
   - Enjoy your food, but eat less.
   - Avoid oversized portions.
2. Foods to Increase
   - Make half your plate fruits and vegetables.
   - Make at least half your grains whole grains.
   - Switch to fat-free or low-fat (1%) milk.
3. Foods to Reduce
   - Compare sodium in foods like soup, bread, and frozen meals, and choose the foods with lower numbers.
   - Drink water instead of sugary drinks.

HOW DOES EXERCISE HELP?

As discussed in Chapter 4, exercise has been shown to be very beneficial to cancer survivors for a number of reasons.

The American Cancer Society, the Centers for Disease Control and Prevention, the World Health Organization, and the American College of Sports Medicine all recommend the following for cancer survivors.

- Exercise at least five times per week.
- Warm up for 5–10 minutes before aerobic activity (such as walking, swimming, or cycling).
- Maintain moderate intensity for 30–45 minutes.
- Cool down for 5–10 minutes at the end of your workout.

Before starting any kind of exercise program, you should check with your healthcare provider that it is safe for you to do so or to learn if you need to take any special precautions. For example, if you have some heart damage from chemotherapy or radiation therapy, this may limit the kind or intensity of exercise you can do. You may want to start by consulting an exercise specialist or physiotherapist to set up a program that is appropriate for you and where you are in your recovery and survivorship stage. It is important that this person understand your history with cancer and the short- and long-term side effects of the cancer and its treatments. It is not enough that the person has training as a personal trainer, as he or she may lack deeper understanding about cancer and the treatment you had, including warning signs to be aware of when working with someone who has had a serious illness.

Try to find a form of exercise, and preferably different kinds of exercise, that you enjoy so that motivation is not a barrier. If you have never enjoyed tennis, now is not the time to force yourself onto the court. Be realistic about your capability, and don't set goals that are too high. Setting unrealistic goals will just end up being a source of frustration and will waste energy instead of creating energy for you. Slow and steady is how you want to approach this, in the beginning at least. You can dream about the Ironman competition, but maybe start training for it next year, or the year after that. Watch your breathing; you should be able to talk while you exercise. If you find that you are breathless, slow down or take a break. Don't set yourself up for failure, as not everyone (or anyone!) can be Lance Armstrong. For most of us, being consistent with getting some form of exercise on a regular basis is as successful as winning the Tour de France. Be mindful of your safety, and do not attempt anything for the first time alone.

Elaine has found that getting Barry to eat properly is a real struggle. She knows that when he's at work, he lives on coffee and the occasional doughnut. She tried years ago to make a healthy lunch for him, but he either left it on the counter or "forgot" to bring the containers home, so she is pretty sure that the homemade lunch was either left to rot in the office refrigerator or thrown away the next day when he found it on his desk or in his briefcase. After the radiation treatments, he was having some problems swallowing, and for a while he lived on Jell-O and applesauce, but now he is able to eat almost everything he ate before. She can see that he is gaining weight—his face is filling out and his clothes don't hang on him—but she is still concerned.

He seems different to her now. He still has not regained his usual energy, and he is even more short-tempered than before. He seems to have lost interest in life, and even phone calls from their daughter, Libby, who is a junior at college, do not cheer him up. Elaine has been searching the Internet for advice on what to do to help him. She keeps reading about the role of exercise for cancer survivors. One night at dinner, she raised the topic. As she expected, the response was not positive.

"What do you mean by 'exercise,' Elaine? I have just enough energy to get through the day—you can surely see how tired I am when I get home? Exactly when am I supposed to do this 'exercise'?"

"Well, we can go for a walk after dinner maybe. It's still light out, and maybe we can just walk around the block or down to the lake."

"How much good is that going to do me? Walking is for . . . old ladies! Maybe if I had the time I could play squash at the club after work, but a walk? No way, no how."

"Well, maybe you could talk to that personal trainer at the club. Jill told me that Rodney has been going to him and is really enjoying working out with him. Could you just try it, for me?" Elaine heard her voice going up and she grimaced. She hated it when she whined, but this was something that she knew would help Barry, and she desperately wanted to help him.

Finding an **exercise partner** is often a wise decision. He or she can motivate you to get out the door when all you want to do is sit on the couch. Think about doing some kind of exercise where a partner is required (ping pong, anyone?) or where the presence of a friend or loved one will make the time go quicker. Sometimes exercise can serve two purposes. For example, yoga takes care of the mind and the spirit. You may find it easier to meditate or do relaxation breathing in conjunction with a yoga practice.

Some cancer centers have **rehabilitation programs** where survivors can exercise under the supervision of rehabilitation specialists, or they may be associated with a gym or facility such as the local YMCA. Although special programs for survivors are great, do not use the lack of such programming as an excuse for not exercising! Research suggests that doing some form of exercise where others are involved tends to be more success- ful than exercising on your own. If you skip a session, someone will call to see where you were. Group motivation, and some- times competition, can go a long way in keeping you active and involved.

It is also helpful to keep track of your **progress**. Many online programs are available in which you enter your activity for the day and a permanent log of your progress is created. Most of these programs can create graphs and charts to show you how well you are doing. You can even go "low tech" and write on a paper calendar—note what kind of exercise you did and for how long every day, and even how you felt while doing it. You will be able to review your progress over time, which can moti- vate you to do more and better.

While you don't have to buy the latest in high-fashion exer- cise clothing, wearing **appropriate gear** can make you feel com- fortable and keep you going. If your feet hurt from wearing old shoes that were not designed for the type of exercise you are doing, you are not likely to want to exercise. Wear clothing in layers so that you can keep your body temperature at a com- fortable level. The most important item of clothing you wear is shoes, so make sure that they are appropriate for the activity you are doing.

Listen to **music** if you find it helps, but be careful about wearing headphones or earbuds when you exercise outside. You need to be able to hear what is going on around you—honking car horns, bicycle bells, children shouting—in case you need to get out of the way or watch out for barriers in your path.

Not everyone loves exercise. If you are one of those people who would rather be doing something else, here are some tips for getting over your **lack of motivation**.

- Promise yourself that no matter how bad you feel, you will do just 10 minutes of exercise. You often will find that once you get going, you will continue beyond the 10 minutes and actually enjoy it and discover the benefit.

- Break down your plan into smaller parts. Start with something that you know you can do, and then do the next part and then the next.

- Figure out what your attitude really is and then work to overcome the negative if that is how you are feeling. Exercise can make you feel better, and when you are feeling good, you are more likely to want to exercise.

- Pick something that you know you can succeed at. Being able to do something increases your confidence, making you more likely to stick to it. That does not mean that you should not challenge yourself to do more; just don't set yourself up for failure by overreaching and disappointing yourself.

- Listen to your family and friends when they encourage (or nag!) you to get out and get moving. They love you and care about your well-being. And if you take them along, they will benefit too.

THE IMPORTANCE OF QUITTING SMOKING

It might seem counterintuitive, but some people continue with bad habits and lifestyle choices, including smoking, after a cancer diagnosis. Studies have found similar smoking rates between cancer survivors (20%) and people without cancer (21%), which means that a significant proportion of survivors continue to smoke after their diagnosis. Younger cancer survivors (18–40 years old) are more likely to report that they smoke than people of the same age without a history of cancer (42.6% versus 26.5%). This suggests that stopping smoking may not be seen as important, or that it is very difficult to do. Smoking often is mentioned as a stress reducer, and perhaps the need to reduce stress supersedes the knowledge that smoking is bad for one's health. It is not unusual to see patients smoking outside healthcare facilities, so even being sick does not seem to reduce the need to smoke. Perhaps in surviving cancer, some people think that they have beaten the odds or have faced the worst, and so they continue to smoke. Having relatives at home who smoke decreases the likelihood that the cancer survivor will quit smoking. Heavy alcohol use is also associated with continued smoking. There have been a limited number of studies looking at what interventions are helpful in assisting cancer survivors to stop smoking. Survivors who continue to smoke may need intensive interventions of different kinds, include counseling, support groups, nicotine replacement in the form of patches, gum, or inhalers, and medication.

Barry didn't see the personal trainer at the club. He soon fell back into drinking too much coffee and eat-

*ing sporadically. And he picked up his other bad hab-
it too: every night when he got home, he poured himself a large whiskey and then had wine with dinner.
He didn't seem to show any effects of the alcohol;
he had been drinking like this ever since he got his
first job, and Elaine knew from her friends that most
of their husbands had one or two drinks in the evening. But he'd had cancer, and she knew the drinking
wasn't good for him, but he was a difficult man to reason with.*

*One night he took his glass of after-dinner brandy
out on the deck. He was out there longer than usual, but Elaine was engrossed in a new program on the
cooking channel and didn't notice how long he'd been
gone. When he came in, she smelled the cigar smoke
even before she saw him.*

*"Barry, have you been smoking?" Her voice went up
at the end of her question, and she felt her throat tight-
en like it always did just before she started to cry.*

*"I can't believe that after all you've gone through
you are still smoking those disgusting cigars! Did having
cancer not teach you ANYTHING?"*

*She didn't even try to stop the tears now. She couldn't
have anyway. She remembered every word that the oncologist had said to them when Barry was first diagnosed. He had explained the link between smoking and
alcohol and the kind of cancer that Barry had. They had
both been shocked that something he thought was actually good for him, the wine, had contributed to the
development of his cancer. At the time, he had sworn*

to her, on Libby's life, that he would not touch anoth-
er cigar and would cut back on the alcohol. But it was
a hollow promise, she now realized. She didn't wait for
him to come up with some rationalization or excuse;
she ran into their bedroom and slammed the door.

Quitting smoking is difficult, more difficult than most people imagine. When asked, 70% of smokers say they want to
quit; 35% try to quit each year, but less than 5% actually quit
for good. Quitting smoking causes significant physical and psychological challenges. You will feel cravings that cause restlessness, headaches, irritability, fatigue, and increased appetite.
These feelings start within hours of your last cigarette, peak at
about 72 hours, and may continue for days and weeks. Often
in the first few weeks you start to feel great—you quit!—and
people around you will compliment you and encourage you
to continue to be tobacco free. But after a while, the novelty
wears off, and that is often when people fall off the wagon and
have "just one" cigarette, which quickly leads to the return to
being a regular smoker.

Many quitting methods are available today, including nicotine patches, inhalers, nasal sprays, and gum, oral medications,
and antidepressants. Many of these are available without a prescription, and so access should not be a barrier. Also, a number
of online support groups and telephone quit lines provide motivation and support. The American Cancer Society (800-ACS-
2345 [800-227-2345] or www.cancer.org) has a lot of information about quitting. The National Cancer Institute also has resources, including a tobacco quit line at 800-QUIT-NOW (800-
784-8669) and a Web site at www.smokefree.gov. People who

use quit lines are twice as likely to be successful than those who try to do it alone.

ALCOHOL

Little research has been done on alcohol use after a cancer diagnosis. Excessive alcohol use is associated with certain kinds of cancer, such as head and neck cancer. Survivors of this kind of cancer are at a fourfold increased risk of a secondary cancer if they continue to drink more than 15 beers a week (just more than two a day). Other studies suggest that adult cancer survivors are unlikely to reduce the amount of alcohol they consume after a cancer diagnosis. Perhaps the link between alcohol intake and the risk of esophageal, bowel, liver, and breast cancer is not that well known in the general population. No studies have evaluated interventions to reduce alcohol use in cancer survivors.

SUN PROTECTION

The link between sun exposure and the development of two kinds of skin cancer is well established; both basal cell and squamous cell cancer, but not melanoma, can be prevented by the use of sunscreen. To date, only one study has been done on the use of sunscreen in cancer survivors, which suggested that using sunscreen lowers sun exposure and the incidence of new cancers. It is recommended that sun protection should be discussed with all cancer survivors as part of rehabilitation after treatment. However, no guidelines exist for this at the present time.

VITAMIN AND MINERAL SUPPLEMENTS

Many claims have been made about the role of vitamin and mineral supplements in cancer prevention. Many of these claims sound too good to be true, and they are. If you eat a balanced diet, you probably do not need to take additional vitamins. But if your diet is lacking, take a good multivitamin every day. As you will read in Chapter 7, prevention of side effects such as osteoporosis calls for daily calcium and vitamin D supplementation at the recommended doses.

Be careful about taking very large doses of any vitamin or mineral. At best, the excess will be excreted in your urine, making for expensive urine, but excess doses of some vitamins can be harmful. Fat-soluble vitamins (A, D, and E) in particular may be stored in the liver or other organs and can do significant damage to your health.

Be very wary about claims of cancer cures from vitamins or minerals. You can be sure that if these claims were true, they would be part of the established treatment protocols for your kind of cancer. Tell your healthcare provider what herbal or natural remedies you are taking because some of them can interact with prescribed medication and be detrimental to your health. There really is not a conspiracy to keep complementary therapies away from cancer survivors. Your oncologist may not know much about these treatments, but your pharmacist can be very helpful in providing information about drug interactions.

WHY IS IT IMPORTANT TO MAKE LIFESTYLE CHANGES?

Making lifestyle changes as described in this chapter can make a big difference in cancer survivors' quality of life. It can help family members and friends, too, if they become involved in the survivor's efforts to live a healthier lifestyle. But these kinds of changes can be hard to make and even harder to maintain. Lifestyle changes require motivation and perseverance to maintain over the long haul. It helps if you don't have to do it alone. The support and encouragement of those you love can go a long way in keeping you motivated and making the changes.

Cancer survivors are able to make significant changes in their lifestyles. One study showed that 92% of cancer survivors did not smoke, and almost 50% did some kind of regular exercise. But less than 20% were eating the recommended minimum servings of fruits and vegetables. And only 5% were meeting all three recommendations for healthy living.

Motivation is important. People who believe that unhealthy behaviors such as smoking, alcohol, or poor diet contributed to their diagnosis of cancer are more likely to make changes to these behaviors and adopt a healthier lifestyle. And survivors who believe that a healthy lifestyle can prevent a recurrence of their cancer also are more likely to institute changes.

After the smoking episode, Elaine and Barry didn't talk for a while. She was really angry with him and felt let down. She knew that if he didn't change, if he continued with his drinking and smoking, that he was at high risk for a recurrence. She was not sure that she could han-

dle that. She seemed to be more affected by his diagnosis than he was. Sure, he was the one who went through the treatment, but she had suffered too. She could remember every drive to the chemotherapy and radiation therapy appointments, how wound up he was and the set of his jaw as he prepared himself for what lay ahead. He had never been one to talk about his emotions, but she could see how he was pushing them down and how he carried his fear in his shoulders and neck. His neck had been so thin when he lost weight, and the radiation had seemed to make it even thinner. And when he was anxious, the muscles of his neck were as taut as guitar strings.

So why wouldn't he try? She understood it was hard to find the time to exercise, and she knew that he was exhausted at the end of every day. And she also knew that he loved his whiskey and wine and after-dinner brandy. But it was not good for him, so why couldn't he just try?

There were days when she just wanted to walk away. Just pack up and go someplace where she didn't have to think and worry about him and the cancer coming back. But she knew that he needed her, and so she pushed those thoughts out of her head. She didn't know what it would take to make him change; she just wished that it would happen.

TAKE-HOME MESSAGES

One of the hallmarks of survivorship is that you have overcome the challenges of treatment and are now on a path of healing and health that will hopefully continue for the rest of your life. Taking good care of yourself and your health is one of the responsibilities of survivorship. Participating in regular exercise has many benefits, including alleviating depression, decreasing fatigue, and improving overall well-being. Coupled with good eating habits, exercise can lead to a more balanced way of living that may protect against recurrence, as well as helping to heal the body and calm the mind. Avoidance of nicotine and limited use of alcohol also are important strategies for good health, and sun protection remains one of the most important cancer prevention interventions.

Making changes to your lifestyle is not easy. Over the span of many years, you have developed habits and ways of living that are comfortable and easy, even enjoyable, for you. Changing those behaviors is challenging, and sustaining them may be even more of an obstacle. Your healthcare providers should be encouraging and helping you to make those changes. Your family and friends may find that supporting you and going along with the changes will provide them with tangible ways of helping you, as well as improving their own health. It's a win-win situation. So get moving and start making the change!

CHAPTER 6

ON HIGH ALERT

M any cancer survivors think they remember every detail of their diagnosis and treatment, but do they? Over time, the stress of those days, weeks, and months and the emotional details may be remembered and the faces of the many healthcare providers may be recalled. But often, survivors and their families forget exactly what tests were done and what treatments were given. There is nothing wrong with this, and it may be a sign of healthy emotional recovery. But there will be times when the survivor needs to know exactly what kind of chemotherapy was given or the details of the tumor that was removed during surgery. How do you do this?

HOW DO YOU REMEMBER THE TREATMENTS?

Some survivors, or their family members, keep precise, detailed notes of every appointment and every blood test or x-ray. These are often filed neatly and in chronological order and kept somewhere safe. Some cancer centers even provide a file where patients can keep these notes. The file usually has print-

ed material explaining the specific cancer that has been diagnosed and the general plan of care. Other families keep the
notes in a box under the desk or in a bookcase and don't do
much with it other than add new results and then ignore what
is jumbled in the box. That is fine too, if that is the way you are
able to cope with the information. What is important is that
you have the information somewhere, that it is organized, and
that you and one or two key family members or support people
can easily access it.

*Stacey was a tiny newborn when her mother, Jen,
noticed something odd about how the light reflected
in her right eye. It just seemed not right. She hoped
she was imagining it, but she took her to the pedia-
trician, and within just a day or two, tiny Stacey was
having surgery for something called retinoblastoma. Jen
could hardly believe what was happening. She and her
partner, Brad, had moved to another town shortly after they got married, and almost as soon as they got
there, Jen found out she was pregnant. She didn't even
bother looking for a job. She was already four months
along, and Brad was old-fashioned that way; he wanted to take care of Jen and the baby. His mom had never
worked outside the home, and that was what he wanted for his family.*

*For years after the surgery, Jen took Stacey for check-
ups every couple of months and then every year. She
had a prosthetic eye made and it needed to be replaced
every couple of years as she grew bigger. By the time
she was 13, she didn't want her mom to go with her to*

appointments, and Jen was afraid that she would skip her appointments. Stacey was getting more and more rebellious, and there were times when Jen hardly knew this tall girl who had replaced her sweet little Stacey.

Cancer survivors who were babies or children when they were diagnosed and treated for cancer have some special needs. Their parents had been through a unique experience when they were too young to have any memory of the disease, which may alter the way their parents treat them. It is common for these parents to overprotect their children both physically and emotionally. Ever since the diagnosis, the parents have had to be very vigilant, especially if the cancer happened when the child was very young and unable to say how he or she was feeling. This overprotective-ness can result in a stormy adolescence as the preteen or teenager tries to be more independent and the parent is unable or too scared to give the child more freedom.

Stacey resisted going to the optometrist more and more. Jen wasn't sure that Stacey was taking good care of her prosthetic eye; she was supposed to keep it meticulously clean, and Jen was so afraid Stacey would get an infection. But if she asked about it, it just resulted in a blowup with Stacey, who had a bad temper, and Jen always ended up in tears. She also started to ask lots of questions about the cancer as she got older. Jen didn't know what or how much to tell her. When she was younger, she had told Stacey that she had a "bad owie" and the doctors had given her a special eye, but she wasn't sure how to talk to Stacey about it now that she was older. A friend of hers, a nurse who worked at the hospital where Stacey had her operation 13 years before, suggested that she show Stacey all her medical records from that time. Jen considered that, and one afternoon she left the box with all of Stacey's medical results on her daughter's bed.

WHAT IS A SURVIVORSHIP CARE PLAN?

In 2006, the Institute of Medicine published a landmark report titled *From Cancer Patient to Cancer Survivor: Lost in Transition.* This report was the first to formally recognize survivorship as a distinct phase of the cancer journey. One key aspect of the report was the recommendation that all members of the healthcare team, the patient, and the family know what treatment was provided, as well as what needed to be done and by whom once that treatment ended.

The report recommended that every patient with cancer receive a written care plan, called the *survivorship care plan* (SCP), that contains at a minimum eight key components.

1. A treatment summary is provided with details of the diagnosis, including the type of cancer, the extent of the disease, and a list of the treatments provided.
2. The care plan includes information about what is to be expected after primary treatment is over.
3. Professional guidelines should be included for other members of the healthcare team for surveillance of recurrence and the development of new cancers.

4. The long-term and late effects of treatment should be described in such a way that the patient understands what might happen and what to look for in the future.
5. Non-cancer-related healthcare needs also should be addressed in this document. These include guidance about diet and exercise, alcohol use, smoking, and immunizations.
6. Psychosocial concerns affect quality of life and are seen as very important and should be addressed in the SCP.
7. Issues about employment, insurance, and other economic issues also may be included.
8. The identification and contact information for all healthcare providers involved in the patient's care should be listed. This needs to be kept up to date so that the right providers can be contacted should the need arise.

The first component, the treatment summary, should include the types of tests performed and the results of these tests. The tumor characteristics should be detailed, including the site of the cancer, the stage and grade, and hormone and receptor marker status. The treatment start and completion dates also should be included. Details should be provided about the type of treatment given (surgery, chemotherapy, radiation, hormonal or endocrine therapy, gene therapy, stem cell or bone marrow transplant), what dosages where given, what, if any, side effects were experienced, and how the patient responded to the treatment.

The next section, what to expect when primary treatment is over, is an important one and something that the survivor and family should pay close attention to. This section of the care plan should explain what to expect during recovery in terms of possible short-term effects from the treatments and what to look for in case of possible recurrence. It also should provide information about possible late effects—complications that can occur many years after treatment, which the survivor may not associate with the original cancer if not warned about it. The care plan also should include whom to contact if anything unexpected happens or if the survivor notices something new, either physically or emotionally, including anticipated short-term and late effects.

The third section recommended for the SCP contains information about guidelines for healthcare providers related to optimum treatment for the particular kind of cancer. Inclusion of this information is recommended so that other healthcare providers and the patient are using the same information. These may become out of date quite quickly as new advances are made, so it should be dated to ensure that future healthcare providers will be aware of whether these guidelines are appropriate. The individual should take the SCP to appointments with the primary care provider so that he or she is fully informed about what has happened and what the suggestions for ongoing care and monitoring are. Do not assume that a copy of the SCP has been provided to the primary care provider; this should happen automatically when the survivor is discharged from the cancer center or hospital, but mistakes do happen. The SCP should include who in the healthcare team is responsible for ordering follow-up investigations and screening.

The next section informs the survivor about what effects to expect. Many survivors are not aware of what to look for regarding long-term side effects, and some may not want to know. Knowing what may happen is important information because not knowing may lead to either ignoring important side effects that can be treated or panicking when something happens and thinking the worst. Knowing about potential problems does not mean that they will happen. The old Boy Scout motto—be prepared—is even more important to cancer survivors than to Boy Scouts!

This book provides you with detailed advice as suggested in section 5 of the SCP. Cancer survivors need to know about staying healthy and living well. This section of the SCP should contain advice about that, as well as information about resources that can be used to help survivors live the best way they can. This section of the SCP may be especially important for survivors of certain kinds of cancer. For example, someone who has survived colon cancer and has an ostomy to collect waste outside the body may need unique information about diet and vitamins to remain healthy when the digestive system is not functioning as before.

Issues such as depression and anxiety, returning to work or school, sexuality and fertility, family coping, and social relationships should be addressed next in the SCP. Cancer affects the whole person and the patient's loved ones, and anticipating life and relationship concerns is important. Once again, it is important for the SCP to contain contact information for service providers such as social workers, psychologists, counselors, and other care providers who deal with emotional and social issues.

Employment and insurance issues become even more important when primary treatment is over. Survivors need to know their rights under the law, as well as the extent and limitation of insurance policies. Information about whom to contact for help with these matters should be provided in section 7 of the SCP.

Section 8 of the SCP is a very important one. This is where contact information for all members of the healthcare team should be entered along with their specialty so that the survivor and the family know whom to contact. This section should be kept up to date with new providers' names entered as they join the healthcare team.

The information in the SCP may be very complex and not something that every cancer survivor wants to know, but it is important information for the future and for other healthcare providers who care for the survivor. The SCP is seen as a living document that is added to over the years and as the needs and developmental stage of the survivor change.

> *Stacey ignored the box for a few days. Then one evening when there was nothing she wanted to watch on TV, she started going through the papers in the box. It was very confusing! She tried to organize the papers into piles, and soon she had a large pile of what looked like blood test results and a smaller pile of letters from the eye specialist to other doctors. There were even some old pictures of her from when she was a baby. She cringed when she saw how awful she looked with her first prosthetic eye. She quickly checked her image in the mirror—she looked way better now. She went back to all the papers and tried to make sense of what they said. After almost two hours, she was still confused. What was her mother thinking when she dumped all of this on her bed?*

WHAT DOES THE SURVIVORSHIP CARE PLAN LOOK LIKE?

Some cancer care providers give the survivor and the family a printed document with all the information from the time of diagnosis through treatment and follow-up. This may be a computer-generated document divided into sections as described previously, or it may be copies of the many tests that have been performed. It can be difficult to interpret these tests and documents, and it is your right to ask for help in understanding what all of this means. Most cancer centers or hospitals will offer the survivor and family an opportunity to go over the documents with a staff member in person, usually a doctor, nurse, or a specialist in survivorship care. This usually happens when the survivor is transitioned out of the cancer care system and back to the primary care provider or into a special survivorship program.

While you are going through treatment or while you are recovering may not be the best time to deal with stacks of paper and test results. You may feel better prepared to do this a little later in your survivorship. However, many survivors just put the documents aside and forget about them! That may be one way of dealing with the whole experience, which is fine as long as you know where the documents are so that you can retrieve them at a future date.

Many cancer care providers give survivors a printed SCP that has been generated by a member of the team and is preferably discussed with the survivor. You can also find care plans online that you can complete yourself using information provided to you by your cancer care team during and after treatment.

The following Web sites provide templates or guidelines for care plans.

- **Journey Forward** (www.journeyforward.org): This Web site provides a template for an SCP that is filled out by your oncology team and then shared with you and your primary care provider. The site also has a library of survivorship resources written for patients.
- **National Comprehensive Cancer Network** (www.nccn.org): This Web site provides evidence-based information and guidelines for your healthcare providers.
- **National Comprehensive Cancer Network for patients** (www.nccn.com): This Web site is for cancer survivors and their supporters. It is a sister site to the one for healthcare professionals and provides up-to-date information for survivors based on the latest evidence.
- **LIVESTRONG Care Plan** (www.livestrongcareplan.org): This tool from LIVESTRONG and OncoLink provides an opportunity to create your own SCP.
- **Prescription for Living** (www.nursingcenter.com/library/static.asp?pageid=721732): This is another template for an SCP that can be completed by your oncology care team.
- **CureSearch Children's Oncology Group** (www.survivorship guidelines.org): This Web site provides guidelines for follow-up care of children and teenagers with cancer.

Stacey's mom asked her about the box of papers about a week later. Reading through all the papers had made Stacey think about what her mom and dad must have gone through when she was a baby and how hard it must have been for them. To her, this was how she had always been—but maybe it was different for them.

"Mom, can I ask you something?" Her voice was hesitant, as though she were afraid of what the answer might be.

"Of course, Stacey. You can ask me anything you want."

"It's about my eye. I mean, it's about what it was like for you when I . . ."

Stacey saw a shadow pass over her mother's face, and she immediately felt bad that she had asked. She started to say something, but Jen interrupted her.

"No, Stacey, I want to talk about this. I've wanted to talk about it for a long time, but I wanted to wait till you were ready. You having cancer . . . it felt like my heart had been torn out of me. I don't know that I have the words for it, but every day since then I have been so thankful that you are here with me, with us, and every day I am proud of you and what you have accomplished."

Stacey ignored the tears that were pouring down her mother's face.

"Mom, I'm not that baby anymore. I want to know everything, and all those papers have kind of made me more confused. Can I talk to the doctors at the cancer center? Maybe they can explain what happened and why."

"Oh, Stacey, I'm not sure that's what's best for you . . ."

But Stacey had stormed out of the room, and Jen heard the front door slam as she left the house.

CHILDHOOD CANCER SURVIVORS

Survivors who had cancer in their childhood present with some unique challenges related to their ongoing care. Because they were too young to remember most of what happened, they rely completely on their parents to inform them about their journey with cancer. Some parents may feel that all of that is in the past and that bringing it up again serves no purpose. Talking about it may be very painful for the parents. They may think that letting go of the past is the best way to deal with the matter. It is common for the parents of a child with cancer to want to control the amount of information given to their child at the time of the cancer and even years later.

As that child grows into a teenager and then a young adult, it is natural for the person to want to know more about the cancer and its treatment, and there are many instances when the individual *needs* to know this information. For example, some children have treatments that are likely to affect their fertility. This is something that they must know before settling into a relationship and planning on starting a family of their own. Challenges to fertility after cancer will be discussed in more detail in Chapter 11. Side effects related to radiation therapy include developmental delays, cognitive challenges, reduced growth, vision and hearing problems from radiation to the head/brain, and cardiac problems if the chest has received radiation. Every system of the body may be affected by exposure to radiation, including the urinary, gastrointestinal, and respiratory systems. If chemotherapy was given, damage to all systems may occur as well. Female childhood cancer survivors appear to experience greater difficulties than their male counterparts and have greater emotional problems as well. The reasons for this are unknown.

Depending on the time since diagnosis, the healthcare team may have changed, as many of the members of the original healthcare team may have moved to other institutions or retired. Old hospital records may have been destroyed or lost, and so constructing a history of past care may be next to impossible. Some late effects of cancer treatment occur decades after the treatment was given, and if survivors do not know the details of their cancer treatment, diagnosing and treating late effects may not happen in a timely manner, if at all.

As these children grow older, most will have a natural curiosity about what happened. Most experts agree that by the time the survivors are young adults, they should know about their cancer history and should take on the responsibility of their own follow-up care. Childhood cancer treatment is a success story: today more than 80% of children diagnosed with cancer go on to survive for years, in comparison to the 1960s when only 28% survived more than five years. But survival comes with a price, and many long-term childhood cancer survivors experience multiple late effects depending on the kind and length of treatment. Most survivors of childhood cancer are well during adolescence and develop health problems later in life. These problems may be secondary cancers caused by radiation therapy or as a result of unique genetic or lifestyle factors. Almost 75% of childhood cancer survivors will develop a chronic disease by the time they are 40 years old, and more than 40% will be diagnosed with a serious health problem.

If survivors do not know the details of their treatment decades ago, or if the records of these treatments are not available to their healthcare providers years later, they may not receive appropriate screening for late effects or recognition that new health problems are related to the distant cancer and its treatment. A study of 635 survivors of childhood cancer revealed that 20 years after their diagnosis, only 72% were able to report their cancer diagnosis accurately and that only 70% of those who received radiation therapy could report the site of the treatment. None of the participants in the study could report a detailed history of the kind of cancer and the specific treatment they were given. Although this may not be surprising given the amount of time that had passed, this does not bode well for their care as adults and into the future, where recall of these factors could influence diagnosis and treatment of late effects.

We don't know exactly what childhood cancer survivors remember about their cancer experience. A study of childhood cancer survivors in their 30s and 40s revealed that these survivors experienced distress and anxiety years later even though they were not totally sure exactly what happened. They are unable to make sense of the experience and, more importantly, to transform the experience into something positive, as many adult survivors are able to do. Because the children did not receive direct explanations when they were young and going through treatment, many have fantasies about what happened that may be worse than the reality.

The next day, Stacey was willing to talk again. Jen told her that she had made an appointment for them to see the original oncologist who had been involved in her treatment 12 years before.

"That's great, Mom, but I want to go alone, okay?"

"Stacey, you can't. You just can't. I know you think you're old enough, but you are 13, and that's not old enough in my eyes. You will just have to live with this decision, young lady."

"Mommmmmm," Stacey's voice dragged into a whine.

"I promise I won't say anything. You can ask all the questions, and I won't say a word unless you ask me to." Jen's voice was firm. What nonsense for a young girl to think she could go see the oncologist all by herself!

Stacey rolled her eyes and flounced back to her room. But she didn't slam the door this time.

It is not all bad, though. Research suggests that many childhood cancer survivors are resilient and thrive in adolescence and adulthood. Young adult cancer survivors report in some studies that they smoke less than their counterparts who have not had cancer and believe that being healthy is especially important for them as cancer survivors. However, in other studies, young adult cancer survivors appear to take risks with their health despite their history.

ADULT CANCER SURVIVORS

SCPs are important for adult survivors, too, for the same reasons that they are important for survivors of childhood cancer. All survivors need a detailed record of the type of cancer they had with details of their treatment. Ideally, this should be a document that the survivors have in their possession and that is updated regularly after follow-up care and shared with all members of their healthcare team, including primary care providers and other specialists outside of the oncology team.

TAKE-HOME MESSAGES

Over and over, experts agree that survivors of childhood cancer need education about their disease and how best to take care of themselves. A comprehensive SCP that is shared with the survivor and healthcare providers outside of the cancer care system is an important step in optimizing care and quality of life. The SCP has eight essential components, including a comprehensive summary of the cancer and its treatment, guidelines for what to look for in the survivorship phase, recommendations for a healthy lifestyle, attention to psychosocial concerns, and a list of contact information for members of the healthcare team.

CHAPTER 7

PROTECTION FOR LIFE

S o you got through treatment, and life should be just plain sailing now, right? Well, unfortunately, that's not the case for many cancer survivors. As the number of survivors continues to grow, we are learning that many of them will experience side effects long after treatment is over. These are called long-term and late effects. *Long-term effects* are those side effects that first appear during treatment and persist after treatment is over; an example of this is fatigue, as discussed in Chapter 4. A *late effect* of cancer treatment is one that was not there during treatment but that appears years later. An example of this is heart problems after radiation to the chest. Compounding these long-term and late effects is the fact that most cancer survivors are older than 65 years old, a time when other chronic diseases, such as diabetes, typically become a problem. These issues are important because they affect the survivor's quality of life and contribute to both physical and psychological functioning in a negative way, decreasing functional and emotional coping at home and at work. Some survivors will have little or no side effects as they live the rest of their lives, while others will be severely burdened. A great deal of variation exists related to the person, the disease, and the treatments.

The risk of developing a second cancer distinct from the original cancer is slightly increased for cancer survivors. This may be the result of genetic and environmental factors associated with the first cancer or because of factors related to the treatment of the first cancer (for example, immune suppression) or generalized genetic susceptibility to cancer.

Stan is 69 years old, and until he was treated for bladder cancer, he felt at least 10 years younger than that. He was diagnosed after a routine visit to his primary care physician, who sent him for a urine test. The result was abnormal, and the next month was filled with more tests and many appointments. Exactly four weeks later, he had surgery to remove the tumor in his bladder. The urologist who did the surgery warned Stan that he might need further treatment because the cancer was aggressive. And that proved to be the case. After the surgery, he had to have six weeks of radiation therapy, which really knocked the wind out of him. And then he had weeks of chemotherapy.

After all this, Stan felt like he was 79 years old! He was weak and tired and had ongoing problems with leakage of urine. He hardly left the house anymore. He was so afraid of having an accident in public, even though his wife, Mona, told him that if he wore the adult diapers, he would be just fine and no one would notice. And he was just so tired that he didn't have the energy to be interested in much. This was not what he imagined his retirement would be like.

WHAT ARE COMMON LONG-TERM AND LATE EFFECTS OF TREATMENT?

The most common long-term effects of cancer therapy are fatigue and depression. Some survivors also report persistent pain. These three often occur together and should prompt intervention. Pain may be related to functional problems caused by joint and muscle changes from treatments including surgery, radiation therapy, and chemotherapy. Fatigue and depression have been described in detail in earlier chapters. Remember that long-term effects start at the time of treatment and then continue for an extended period of time afterward. Other long-term effects of cancer treatment are the following.

- Sexual problems (see Chapter 10) and urinary problems such as leakage or the frequent need to urinate are also common after treatment to the pelvis or abdomen.
- Diarrhea is a common long-term effect of both surgery and radiation to the bowel after treatment for colon cancer and prostate cancer.
- Some kinds of chemotherapy result in changes in sensation of the feet and hands, which may result in difficulties with balance and walking. Other survivors experience dry mouth and long-term dental problems as a result of chemotherapy.
- Women who have had radiation to the pelvis for the treatment of uterine, cervical, or vulva cancer frequently experience vaginal dryness, which may lead to both sexual and relationship problems.
- Women who receive chemotherapy may experience persistent absence of menstrual periods. The chemotherapy stops the ovaries from producing hormones. Some women may

see the return of their normal menstrual cycle (particularly younger women; however, it is dose and agent dependent), whereas women closer to the usual age for menopause may never have a period again.

- Some treatments (for example, the endocrine therapies called *aromatase inhibitors* used to prevent recurrence of breast cancer) also increase the survivor's risk for the development of osteoporosis.

- Long-term use of steroids increases the risk of destruction of bone, particularly in the hips.

- Some survivors report cognitive changes that begin during treatment and persist for years afterward. This is discussed in detail in Chapter 8.

- Stem cell and bone marrow transplant survivors may be at increased risk for chronic infections because of the need for immune-suppressive therapy to prevent graft-versus-host disease.

Patients with cancer should be warned about the potential for long-term effects *before* they start treatment, and this information should be repeated multiple times as they go through treatment and in follow-up care. We are never sure exactly what information our patients are hearing, absorbing, and remembering, so repetition is necessary. However, many health-care providers have a mental checklist of what they need to tell patients. Even if they provide this information at a time when the patient cannot take in the information, once they have done it, they tick it off their mental checklist and don't talk to the patient about it again. Survivors are often reluctant to ask about something again or for additional information. They don't want to appear to be stupid or disrespectful when

they know or think they know that they have been told something already.

> *Five years later, Stan received a clean bill of health
> from the urologist. His children and grandchildren were
> overjoyed and insisted on taking him out to his favor-
> ite steakhouse for a celebration dinner. How could he
> tell them that this was the last thing he felt like doing?
> Even though he was theoretically cured—five years after
> treatment with no signs of recurrence, as the doctor ex-
> plained—he felt awful most of the time. He had the oc-
> casional good day, or if he was really lucky he had a string
> of two or three good days, but in general he felt crap-
> py. There was no other way to describe it. He had men-
> tioned to the doctor that he needed to urinate often, but
> the doctor just told him to restrict fluids starting in the
> late afternoon, and that was that. Stan didn't tell him that
> he was still having leakage, and he was sick and tired
> of wearing those awful diapers if he wanted to go out
> for any length of time. Golf had become almost impossi-
> ble, and he missed his old friends from the golf club. He
> missed feeling normal too—and the odd erection would
> be nice, come to think of it! Those had disappeared right
> after his surgery five years ago, seemingly never to return.
> If this was living, he was not sure he wanted it.*

Late Effects of Surgery

Late effects of cancer treatment occur many months or years
after treatment is over and weren't there when treatment end-

ed. Stan is experiencing late effects of his treatment regimen with an increased need to urinate frequently. This is in addition to the leakage that started during or soon after his surgery. The need to urinate more frequently may be as a result of his bladder shrinking in response to the radiation, which may be made worse by scarring of the bladder from chemotherapy. Or his bladder may be smaller after the tumor was removed, and so he needs to empty it more frequently.

Late effects of surgery are dependent on the site of the surgery and include pain and cosmetic changes that can have far-reaching effects on self-image and self-esteem. The pain may be at the site of the wound or scar, or it may be internal and caused by scar tissue and damage to nearby organs. The following are some specific late effects of surgery related to the surgical site.

- Cognitive changes may result if the surgery involved the brain or spinal cord. Survivors may notice changes in sensation and movement of limbs, as well as changes in vision, hearing, and language, depending on where in the brain the tumor was located.
- Survivors of surgery to the head and neck may notice difficulties with speech, swallowing, and breathing along with changes to the way that facial and neck muscles function, resulting in altered facial appearance and expression.
- Many years after surgical removal of lymph nodes anywhere in the body, swelling can occur in the arm, leg, or other areas from where lymph drains. This swelling may be cosmetically challenging and also may affect movement.
- Surgery to the bowel or other abdominal organs may result in alterations in bowel functioning, as well as pain and increased risk of internal obstruction.

- Pelvic surgery commonly causes infertility and sexual difficulties such as erectile dysfunction, inability to have an orgasm, and loss of ejaculation. Incontinence is also possible, as are internal obstructions caused by the presence of scar tissue adhering to the bowel.

- Amputation of limbs, hands, or feet may result in alterations in body image and self-esteem, as well as functional limitations that affect activities of daily living and the ability to work. Survivors of amputation often experience phantom pain and sensation where the limb used to be. Amputation also increases the risk of arthritis in other joints because of the need to compensate for the missing limb.

- Survivors who had surgery to remove a tumor or tumors in the lungs often experience shortness of breath, loss of energy, and generalized weakness. This leads to very poor quality of life.

- Men who had their prostate removed to treat prostate cancer usually survive for many years, but those years are often of poor quality as the men commonly experience urinary incontinence, erectile difficulties, and diminished masculine self-image. Ongoing problems with incontinence may result in social isolation and poor health related to a sedentary lifestyle because the survivors don't get regular exercise because of fear of leakage.

- Younger women who had their ovaries removed experience premature menopause and loss of fertility. This can cause a great deal of suffering and even relationship breakdown.

- Men who had a testicle surgically removed, often for the treatment of testicular cancer, may experience loss of or reduced fertility and loss of masculine self-image. For men who had both testicles removed for the treatment of prostate cancer (called an *orchiectomy*), testosterone deficiency may result. This causes loss of energy, weight gain, depression and irritability, erectile dysfunction and loss of sexual desire, muscle loss, hot flashes, sleep disturbance, and an increased risk for the development of diabetes and cardiovascular disease.

• Survivors of colorectal cancer who had part or all of their bowel or rectum removed usually have an ostomy created where their waste is collected in a bag on the outside of the body. This can result in poor body image, as well as loss of appetite, internal obstruction, and hernia development.

Late Effects of Radiation Therapy

Survivors who have been treated with radiation therapy are at increased risk for secondary cancer anywhere in the body, which usually occurs about 10 or more years after treatment for the primary cancer. Other late effects of radiation therapy include the following.

• Damage to bones can lead to deformities, breakage, and bone destruction, causing functional disability and pain.

• Radiation to the chest can lead to damage to the heart and major blood vessels. This damage can be in the form of scarring of the heart muscle or the sac surrounding the heart (the pericardium). Or it can cause inflammation of the heart itself or the large vessels leading into and out of the heart. The blood vessels supplying the heart itself also may be damaged, causing the heart to function abnormally.

• Radiation to the chest or lungs can also cause scarring of the lungs and decreased ability to function, leading to severe shortness of breath and diminished energy.

- Radiation to the head and neck can cause problems with the endocrine system, resulting in hormone imbalances and leading to sterility. It can also cause problems in the mouth, leading to extreme dryness and eventual dental problems.
- Radiation to the face and brain also can cause significant damage to the eyes; cataracts, dry eyes, and vision loss may result.
- Radiation to the brain results in cognitive and personality changes, difficulties with memory and learning, and potentially changes to the structure of the brain that can cause widespread effects, depending on where in the brain the damage has occurred.
- Radiation to the abdomen can cause internal blockages if the bowel becomes damaged. The bowel tissues are very susceptible to radiation damage, and chronic diarrhea or constipation also may result.
- Other internal organs such as the liver and kidneys can be damaged and result in chronic health problems, such as liver failure or high blood pressure in the case of kidney damage.
- If lymph nodes are the target of radiation therapy or are in the radiation field, damage may result in blockage of lymph drainage. Lymphedema (swelling) may result, with the same consequences as those occurring after surgical removal of the lymph nodes.
- Radiation to the pelvis that includes the bladder and bowel may result in changes in the structure or size and capacity of the bladder.
- Skin changes, including loss of hair and thinning of the skin, are also common in the area where the radiation beam was aimed.

Late Effects of Chemotherapy and Hormonal Therapy

Although the acute effects (those that develop at the time that the chemotherapy is being given) of chemotherapy are well known, globally screened for, and mostly able to be treated or prevented, knowledge about late effects is really in its infancy. As survivors live longer and longer after initial treatment, we are discovering more about the late effects. However, treatment for these lags behind. The following are the most common late effects of chemotherapy and hormonal therapy. Many are similar to radiation therapy late effects, but some are different.

- The risk of secondary cancer elsewhere in the body is increased in those who have used steroids, alkylating agents, and anthracyclines.
- Steroids can cause degeneration of bone with an increased risk of fractures.
- Steroids also increase the risk of developing diabetes years after treatment and can cause the development of cataracts in the eyes.
- Inflammation of heart muscle and congestive heart failure may occur after treatment with taxanes, anthracyclines, and high-dose cyclophosphamide.
- Alkylating agents are also responsible for ovarian and testicular shutdown with subsequent loss of fertility and other symptoms of premature menopause in women and testosterone deficiency in men. This may result in loss of sexual desire, pain with sexual activity, inability to achieve sexual satisfaction, and eventual relationship problems.
- Methotrexate and multiagent chemotherapy regimens may lead to damage to the brain causing memory changes, problems with learning, paralysis, and seizures. Cisplatin causes

changes in sensation (numbness and tingling), and hearing loss is also possible.

- Drugs such as bleomycin and methotrexate can cause scarring of the lungs and decreased functioning of the lungs. Some drugs (gemcitabine, for example) may make the effects of radiation to the lungs more severe.

- Some chemotherapy drugs cause long-term damage to the bladder, resulting in urinary frequency, bleeding, urgency, and pain with urination.

- Androgen deprivation therapy, commonly achieved with long-term use of drugs that shut down production of testosterone, causes weakness and fatigue, hot flashes, erectile dysfunction, loss of libido, irritability, cognitive changes, increased risk for diabetes and cardiovascular disease, weight gain, and loss of muscle mass. These are similar to the effects of surgical removal of the testicles.

- Steroids and methotrexate can cause immune suppression and impaired immune function, leaving the survivor susceptible to infections that may be life threatening.

Stan continued to feel crappy, as he described it. He couldn't remember the last time he felt well. He tried as best he could to find the energy to spend time with his grandchildren. They were now teenagers, almost young adults, and he was thankful that they didn't want to play rough like they used to when they were younger. He was surprised when he received a letter from the urologist who had treated his bladder cancer telling him that his care was being transferred back to his primary care provider, Doc Simons. Included with the let-

ter was a summary sheet with the details of his treatment. He read it over and over. It looked so innocent—just black letters on white paper. Not at all like the gray that his life had become. He wasn't sure why he'd received this document. He placed it in a desk drawer, next to his will and important insurance papers.

Later that summer, he slipped on loose gravel when he got out of the car in the supermarket parking lot. Mona made the most terrible fuss, and it seemed like everyone stopped what they were doing and stared at him as he sat on the ground. This made him madder than a snake, and he refused to go to the urgent care center. He insisted that they forget the shopping and go straight home. His hip hurt worse than ever—a deep, dull ache that occasionally flared into white-hot agony if he moved suddenly. He managed to live with it for almost two weeks, but one morning he just couldn't bear it and he asked Mona to drive him to see Doc Simons. He didn't have an appointment, but the receptionist saw the pain in his face and told him that Dr. Simons' younger colleague could see him in about 20 minutes if he could wait. Dr. Simons was fully booked the whole morning, so it was either Dr. Green or the emergency department. Stan decided to take his chances with the new guy, and he waited. Dr. Green turned out to be in his 40s and was very efficient. He sent Stan for an x-ray immediately after listening to his story. Within the hour, Stan found out that he had a hairline fracture of his hip, right where the thighbone fit into the socket. How on earth had this happened?

HOW CAN THESE LATE EFFECTS BE PREVENTED?

It may not be possible to avoid most of the late effects, as the treatment is necessary to deal with the cancer. What is very important is that cancer survivors and their healthcare providers are educated to recognize the signs of late effects of all the treatments given and screen for them as part of follow-up care. Late effects can develop slowly over the years following active treatment, and the survivor may become used to the symptoms and accommodate any functional changes. For example, memory loss may be assumed to be part of the normal aging process. The survivor and family may not be aware of how many changes have occurred in daily life and functioning and how they have all adapted to the changes. Oftentimes the late effects may not be noticed until something serious happens, like Stan's hairline fracture of his hip, which likely occurred as a late effect of the radiation to his bladder and perhaps the chemotherapy weakening his bones as well. But do the survivor and healthcare provider link the distant treatment with the injury or new illness? This may depend on their level of knowledge about what treatments were given long ago and what late effects are associated with the specific treatments.

WHICH LATE EFFECTS CAN BE MINIMIZED OR PREVENTED?

Certain late effects can be prevented in part. These include osteoporosis, diabetes, cardiovascular disease, and dental problems. The risk for certain secondary cancers can be decreased by participating in a healthy lifestyle and avoiding known car-cinogens (substances that are known to cause cancer).

It is well known that many cancer survivors are highly moti-vated to make changes to their lifestyle in the hopes that their health can be preserved as much as possible. For example, studies have shown that 15%–30% of cancer survivors increase their level of physical activity after the cancer diagnosis. Be-tween 40% and 72% increase the amount of fruits and vege-tables in their diet and lower the amount of fat that they eat. Breast cancer survivors are more likely to have screening tests for cervical cancer (Pap smears) and colorectal cancer (fecal occult blood test or colonoscopy) than women without a can-cer history. This may be because these women are connected to the healthcare system because of their cancer. But sustain-ing these changes in the long term may be more difficult. It may be that survivors who experience more late effects and are being treated for them and other chronic conditions may be more connected to the healthcare system and therefore re-ceive more screening and care, whereas relatively healthy sur-vivors may have less contact with the healthcare system and re-ceive less screening and preventive care.

A recent study of cancer survivors reported that 78% had a routine physical checkup, 66% had visited a dentist, and 54% had an influenza vaccination in the previous year. Eighty per-cent of the sample did not smoke, 52% participated in some form of physical activity, and 37% maintained a healthy weight. However, only 31% received all three of the clinical services mentioned previously, and only 16.5% participated in all three healthy lifestyle practices. Participation in the first three ac-tivities (routine checkup, dental care, and influenza vaccination) was more common for those older than 40 years and for those who had diabetes. Being separated or divorced and experiencing poorer mental health lowered the participation rate for these three activities. Factors that increased the chances of healthy lifestyle practices (not smoking, physical activity, and healthy weight) included being female, being older than 65 years, and having a high school education. Factors that decreased healthy lifestyle practices included being of African American race, being separated or divorced, having diabetes, and being depressed.

Osteoporosis can be prevented in part by performing regular weight-bearing exercise, increasing dietary intake of calcium-rich foods, and taking a daily calcium supplement with vitamin D. Regular bone density monitoring can identify those at higher risk, and a number of treatments are available (called *bisphosphonates*) that can increase bone density.

Diabetes can be prevented in part by maintaining a healthy body weight, getting regular exercise, not smoking, and regularly screening blood glucose levels to identify early signs of impaired glucose metabolism.

Cardiovascular disease can be prevented in part by identifying cancer survivors who have received agents with known cardiac effects or radiation therapy to the chest and monitoring them carefully for the earliest signs of cardiac problems. Regular checks of blood pressure and cholesterol levels will indicate survivors with changes suggestive of cardiac damage. Additional testing can be provided to help diagnose and treat any disease as early as possible. Other risk reduction strategies include not smoking and maintaining a healthy weight.

Dental caries can be prevented with regular dental care before and after radiation treatment and chemotherapy known to cause dry mouth. Regular dentist visits, daily use of fluoride mouthwashes, drinking fluoridated water, and exemplary brushing and flossing will all help to reduce the risk of dental caries secondary to lack of saliva after treatment.

The hairline fracture was a turning point for Stan. He saw Dr. Green regularly while the fracture healed. He had to use crutches and take it easy. Over time the pain went away, and on x-ray the fracture was getting better. Dr. Green went through the treatment summary with Stan, explaining the importance of them both understanding the risks of the treatment he had received and being proactive in making changes to his lifestyle that would prevent further illness or injury. He asked Stan about his diet and exercise habits and shook his head when Stan admitted to enjoying a daily cigar on the back porch after dinner. The nightly glass of red wine could stay, but the cigars had to go. Stan smiled sheepishly and nodded. Mona would be completely supportive of this change, of that he was sure.

TAKE-HOME MESSAGES

Long-term and late effects pose a significant threat to the well-being and longevity of cancer survivors. All kinds of treatments can cause these effects. Long-term effects are those that start during treatment and persist long after treatment is over, whereas late effects start long after treatment is over. Both the survivor and the survivor's healthcare providers need to know about the potential for late effects in particular, as these often are not considered to be a consequence of the distant treatment for cancer. Some survivors ignore or adapt to changes in health status and do not report these changes, thus delaying diagnosis and treatment. A detailed summary of treatment, such as a survivorship care plan, is a useful guide for both the survivor and healthcare providers and can serve as a reminder of what side effects to be aware of, even years after treatment is over.

CHAPTER 8

IN A FOG

F or many years, cancer survivors have been telling their healthcare providers that after treatment, their thinking was not as clear as it used to be. Some were told that it was all in their heads (yes, that's exactly where it is!), while others were told that they should just be grateful to be alive. Healthcare providers were not sure that any specific condition really existed and were also not sure what caused it: Was it the cancer itself? Or perhaps it was the chemotherapy, but which specific agent or combination of drugs? Or maybe it was a manifestation of depression or anxiety or a symptom of menopause in women. It was also minimized because most survivors adapted to any changes they were experiencing, but some did have lifelong problems in their jobs and relationships. Another challenge was that there was no clear way of diagnosing it, preventing it, or treating it. So it was largely ignored or attributed to something else.

In more recent years, cancer specialists, psychologists, and others have shown increased interest in this phenomenon, which was first called *chemobrain* or *chemo fog* and is now referred to as cancer- or cancer treatment–associated cognitive changes. It is estimated that between 75% and 95% of

cancer survivors show some signs of cognitive changes shortly after the completion of treatment, and 17%–35% of survivors still have challenges two or more years after treatment
is over.

> *Joan is a teacher who was diagnosed with breast
> cancer at the age of 52 after a routine mammogram.
> The diagnosis came as a complete shock, as there was
> no history of cancer in her family at all. Her relatives ei-
> ther died of a heart attack or stroke at an early age (her
> father's siblings) or they lived well into their 80s. Her
> parents were both alive and well and living in Phoe-
> nix, and her siblings, all three older than her, were ac-
> tive and healthy.*
>
> *She had a mastectomy with reconstruction within
> two weeks of her diagnosis. Her recovery was slow-
> er than she expected, and she was not feeling all that
> great when she started chemotherapy. But she got
> through six months of that and then started what they
> called "hormone therapy," which had been explained
> to her as medication to reduce her risk of a recurrence
> by removing all the estrogen in her body.*
>
> *Her friends all commended her on the way she
> had accepted the diagnosis and moved through treat-
> ment. "What's to be commended?" she wondered. "I
> feel horrible, I look horrible, and my brain's not work-
> ing like it used to." Her family—her husband, Brent, in
> particular—had noticed that ever since her diagnosis,
> something had changed about her. She just seemed . . .
> fuzzy.*

WHAT CAUSES CANCER-RELATED COGNITIVE CHANGES?

The cause of these cognitive changes is a topic of much debate and investigation. For those with brain cancer, changes in cognition and daily functioning are likely to be linked to structural changes after surgery, radiation therapy, or medications that directly target the tumor and tissue nearby. But what about other kinds of cancer? We know that women with breast cancer who are treated with surgery alone also experience cognitive changes. These are often attributed to anxiety and depression or to preexisting changes that have gone unnoticed by the patient and her family. Perhaps some of the changes after surgery can be related to the anesthesia, but this should resolve quickly as the anesthetic agents are cleared by the body.

Changes after chemotherapy are thought to be associated with toxic effects of the medication on brain and nervous tissue, microscopic damage to blood vessels in the brain, release of stress hormones, changes to the cells in the brain brought about by prolonged stress, and the release of *cytokines*, which are proteins involved in communication between cells and that are known to cause inflammation in the brain. Much still needs to be learned about the causes of cognitive changes in cancer survivors, and new knowledge is being generated and learned every day.

Evidence shows that medications that control the amount of sex hormones (estrogen in women and testosterone in men) have an effect on cognition and mental functioning. Estrogen is known to be protective of cognitive functioning, especially in the area of verbal memory. Women who have estrogen receptor–positive breast cancer (about 75% of patients) are usually prescribed drugs such as tamoxifen (a selective estrogen receptor modifier) or aromatase inhibitors (such as letrozole and anastrozole) to limit estrogen in the tissues of the body and reduce the risk of recurrence. These medications have been shown to affect cognitive functioning, with the aromatase inhibitors affecting functioning more than tamoxifen does. Given that women will take these drugs for 5–10 years following their diagnosis, these effects are concerning.

Men with prostate cancer may be prescribed drugs (known as LHRH agonists, or luteinizing hormone-releasing hormone agonists) to reduce the amount of testosterone their body produces and thus limit the growth of cancer cells. These men also experience cognitive changes, and many men stay on the medication for years after diagnosis.

WHAT DO CANCER-RELATED COGNITIVE CHANGES LOOK AND FEEL LIKE?

Cognitive changes can occur anywhere along the cancer trajectory from the time of diagnosis, through active treatment, and then into the survivorship phase. The changes are usually subtle. Some survivors manage to mask them or adapt so that the changes are less noticeable. However, when the changes persist over time or worsen, or when there is a definite pattern, these changes are likely due to something other than chance or lack of sleep.

These cognitive changes have many manifestations:

• Inability to concentrate

- Lack of focus or attention
- Forgetfulness
- Changes to visual memory (not remembering where you put something)
- Decreased mental clarity (feeling fuzzy)
- Mental confusion
- Trouble remembering details, names, and common words
- Difficulty multitasking and finishing certain tasks
- Not being able to learn new skills
- Decreased fine motor dexterity
- Slower thinking and processing
- Decreased ability to make decisions
- Fatigue.

At the time of diagnosis, some survivors find that they are unable to concentrate and are forgetful. This may be associated with the shock of receiving a life-threatening diagnosis as well as the anxiety that accompanies the uncertainty about the days, weeks, and months to come. Sleep disturbances are common after a cancer diagnosis, and cognitive changes may be blamed on lack of sleep and feeling exhausted.

In the months after her surgery and chemotherapy, Joan spent a lot of time alone at home. Brent, her husband, traveled three days a week for his job, and their two kids, Becky and Jon, were away at college and couldn't come home that often. The doctors had advised her to stay home as long as she could, and the principal at her school was supportive and encouraged her to take all the time she needed before coming back. But she was bored and lonely, and so, two months to the day after her last chemo treatment, she went back to her classroom.

She was nervous about what the kids would say and how they would act. Eighth-grade students can be surprisingly mature or immature in her experience. But, they seemed happy to see her and were eager to tell her how useless the substitute teachers had been. The first day nearly wiped her out; she'd forgotten how noisy and energetic a room full of 14-year-olds could be. But day by day her stamina returned, and after a month, she didn't need to take a nap when she got home at 4 pm.

When she had been back for about six weeks, Gary, the principal, asked to see her during one of her breaks. She thought nothing of his request until she saw his face when she sat down across from him.

"Joan, this is not easy . . ."

Her heart contracted and an icy chill went down her spine. She held her breath as he continued.

"I have some concerns about your performance since your return. I've had some complaints from three or four of the parents—"

"What kind of complaints? Things have been fine." Joan's voice was shaky as she interrupted him.

"Calm down, Joan. It's not about class; well, at least the complaints are not about what's happening in the classroom. It seems that homework assignments have not been returned to the kids, and also about some grades for in-class work."

Joan stared at him in confusion. What was he talking about? Her mind whirled as she tried to recall what

homework assignments she had given and what grades
she had awarded.

"I'm going to have to institute some changes in your
assignment, Joan. Just in the interim while we get to
the bottom of this. I've asked Pat Sullivan to come in as
a second teacher in your class. She knows your class,
as she substituted for you while you were off. She'll be
there to help you."

Joan's eyes filled with tears and she jumped out of the
chair and left the office before she started to cry out loud.

It is difficult to have insight into our own behavior and the
subtle changes that have occurred. As human beings we are
very good at adapting to maintain the status quo. The adap-
tations we make can be so effective that not even our closest
family members notice any changes. It can be very difficult for
family and friends to talk about changes they see in us, so they
often pretend that nothing is wrong or make excuses for the
changes they see. "She's so tired, that's why she's forgetting
things," or "He's been through so much; it's no wonder he gets
a bit confused at times."

Joan went home in tears. She sat in her car for a while
when she reached her house and tried to remember
what mistakes she could have made. She wasn't aware
of the time passing and was surprised when Brent's car
pulled into the driveway and he parked behind her.

"Honey, what's wrong? Why are you sitting here?
Are you okay?" Brent's voice echoed the worried look
on his face.

Joan opened her mouth to tell him what had happened at school, but no words came out, just great sobs. Brent helped her out of the car and into the house. He poured them both a glass of wine and waited for her to stop crying long enough to tell him what was going on. He listened with great concentration and then in his usual can-do manner told her that she needed to see her doctors immediately to find out what was wrong. Joan just nodded. It felt good to have him take charge. But she was still very scared.

ARE THERE TESTS TO FIND COGNITIVE CHANGES?

Some tests are able to identify specific areas of mental functioning that have been affected after treatment. However, no definitive test exists that will tell doctors if a survivor has cancer-related cognitive changes. Neuropsychologists are the experts in the use and interpretation of these tests and would usually be the ones who administer them to the survivor. There are special tests that assess attention, concentration, information processing and speed, language, motor function, learning, memory (visual and verbal), visuospatial skills, and executive functioning (decision making). The results of these tests can provide information about where in the brain there is a problem, but they do not give information about the cause or the association with cancer treatments. Many of the cognitive changes associated with cancer treatments are too subtle to be picked up by these tests, which have been developed to identify people with brain injury and developmental problems. Completing the many tests to measure the various aspects of cognition can take from four to eight hours, and this poses a significant challenge itself. The results also do not provide suggestions for treatment of any deficits and have not been validated in large studies of cancer survivors.

The diagnosis of cancer-related cognitive changes is made based on the description of the survivor and family of the changes they have seen and the losses incurred by the survivor. These descriptions usually are more sensitive and accurate in identifying the very subtle changes that typically are experienced.

That night after she had been called into the principal's office, Joan and Brent searched the house to find any papers or work that her students had completed and that she had lost. There was nothing in the home office and nothing in the kitchen where she usually marked their work. She opened and closed the kitchen drawers over and over until eventually Brent snapped at her that the noise was making him crazy. After an hour of fruitless searching, they called it quits and had dinner. Joan picked at the food on her plate and Brent was so deep in thought that he finished his meal without tasting a morsel. The next morning when Brent opened the cabinet under the sink to find a new tube of toothpaste, he found a folder with the missing papers. What were they doing under the bathroom sink?

Joan saw her oncology specialist a week later. Brent canceled a business trip to go with her, and she was glad that he was with her. She was terrified that they were going to tell her that she had Alzheimer disease or permanent brain damage and that she could no longer teach. She hardly slept the week before her appointment. Her sleep had not been good for a while because of the hot flashes that made her pour with sweat, but now she lay awake at night, thinking and worrying about what was wrong with her.

The oncologist asked lots of questions. As Brent heard Joan struggle to answer them, he found himself adding his observations of the changes in her behavior. It hurt him to see her reaction to what he told the doctor. She seemed to shrink in the chair and her shoulders dropped with every statement he made about the changes he had seen in her. It surprised him too—why had he not spoken up before this?

WHAT TREATMENTS CAN HELP WITH COGNITIVE CHANGES?

There is no magic bullet to treat the cognitive changes associated with cancer and its treatments. Because this condition is so common, it has been suggested that patients should be warned about the potential for alterations in cognition **before** they start treatment, as some people may refuse treatment based on this information. This approach has not received much support among cancer doctors, and so most patients are not informed before treatment.

It is important that the survivor and family be told that these cognitive changes are not associated with other conditions, such as Alzheimer disease, and also that this is not a sign of recurrence or associated with an increased risk of the cancer coming back. It can be very reassuring to the survivor and family to know that the changes are linked to treatment, that they are common among survivors, and that the survivor is not going crazy. This reassurance alone can be of great benefit.

Strategies such as the following have been used with older adults experiencing cognitive changes and can be helpful for cancer survivors with specific identifiable challenges.

- Make written reminders of tasks that need to be done. It is important, however, to remember WHERE these reminders are kept! Many people complain about this—making lists and then forgetting to take the list with them or forgetting where the list is. This may be a part of our busy lives as well as a sign of forgetfulness associated with the cancer.

- If you are having trouble with complex tasks, it may be helpful to break down the task into smaller actions and to make a list of these. You then follow the actions on the list one by one until you have accomplished the task. You may need some help in breaking down the task, especially if you are having difficulty understanding complex tasks.

- Program your smart phone or digital diary to remind you to do something at the right time. These electronic devices sound an alert at the time that you need to do the task. However, being able to learn how to program the device may be challenging to survivors who are having difficulty learning new skills. Much like the other electronic devices in our lives today, asking a young person to do it may save a lot of frustration in trying to learn a new skill.

- Keep track of appointments or events on a large calendar using sticky notes. Every day you then remove the sticky note and place it somewhere you will be sure to find it (on the outside of your wallet, for example, or the dashboard of your car) and then you have a mobile reminder of what you are supposed to do.

- You can also record reminders of what you need to do using the recording app in your smart phone. Of course, you then need to remember to listen to your recording and to bring your smart phone with you!

> *Joan asked the oncologist repeatedly for a pill or something that would help.*
>
> *"I have to keep my job. If I can't teach, I don't know what I will do. I'd go crazy for sure! I've worked all these years, even when the kids were growing up, and not having my work would kill me. Life would not be worth living."*
>
> *The oncologist looked at Joan for a while before speaking.*
>
> *"Joan, do you think you're depressed?"*
>
> *"Of course I'm depressed! How would you feel if your boss told you that you were doing a lousy job?"*
>
> *"Of course, I understand that. But do you think you were depressed before this happened at school?"*
>
> *Joan didn't answer immediately. She didn't know. Most of what had happened during treatment was a blur to her, and the past few weeks were shrouded in exhaustion and, more recently, worry.*
>
> *"I'd like you to see our psychologist," the doctor said. "And perhaps the occupational therapist can offer*

some advice about work issues. There really is no pill I can give you, but if you're depressed, we can treat that and see if things improve."

Some evidence has shown that a drug called methylphenidate (Ritalin®) can be helpful in treating cancer-related cognitive changes. It is a psychostimulant and is used in the treatment of attention-deficit/hyperactivity disorder. It has shown some benefit in women with breast cancer. However, like all medications, it has side effects, and survivors need to decide whether they want to risk these effects.

Because the use of drugs that lower levels of estrogen have been implicated in the development of cognitive changes, some women stop taking them for a time to see if that helps. This is a difficult decision for the woman to make. The fear of recurrence may be so strong that it is unthinkable to stop taking something that could lower the risk of the cancer coming back. A discussion with the treating oncologist about the risks of stopping the medication and what that means to recurrence is important.

Two weeks later, Joan saw the psychologist. He asked her lots of questions about her mood and energy levels, and then told her that taking an antidepressant may help her. She looked at her list of questions that she had made before she came to the appointment.

"What are the side effects of these pills?"

"Well, you may have some changes in your sleep pattern and some other side effects, but these usually go away after three or four weeks."

Joan thought for a few minutes, and responded, "I don't think I want to take more pills. Is there anything else I can do?"

ALTERNATIVES TO MEDICATION

If the survivor has depression along with cognitive changes, cognitive-behavioral therapy can be very helpful. It is very important to identify whether the survivor really is depressed before starting this kind of counseling. Cognitive-behavioral therapy is discussed in detail in Chapter 3.

The following week, Joan had her appointment with the occupational therapist. This appointment went much better than the one with the psychologist. Her name was Lilly, and she asked lots of questions about Joan's work and energy levels. She also asked about what Joan was doing to help herself. Joan had to laugh at that—she was mostly feeling bad about herself and had been unable to drag herself out of a spiral of guilt and feeling stupid. She told Lilly about the substitute teacher who came to the classroom every day. Even though she was a nice woman and a good teacher who the kids seemed to like, Joan couldn't help feeling like she was a bad student who needed a remedial teacher herself!

"And how much exercise are you getting, Joan?"

"Uh, nothing. Between work and feeling exhausted, I really don't feel like it. It's all I can do to get dinner

together, and that's only when my husband is home. If
he's away, I have a bowl of cereal and drop into bed."

Exercise has been effective in helping survivors with cognitive changes. As you have read in Chapter 5, regular exercise has many benefits for cancer survivors. Yet another is that exercise promotes oxygen flow to the brain and may combat some of the changes associated with this condition. It also improves strength, stamina, and energy levels, allowing for the brain to concentrate on the task at hand instead of trying to stay awake.

Other strategies to help increase concentration are to limit background noise (for example, switching off the TV or radio when you are trying to do work that requires focus) and to avoid multitasking (such as marking papers while trying to cook dinner). Doing intellectually stimulating activities (Sudoku anyone?) and crossword puzzles also can help to maintain brain flexibility.

It is also important to optimize both the amount and quality of sleep. Being tired all the time reduces your ability to think clearly and concentrate, multiplying the effects of any cognitive challenges you face. Although taking sleeping pills may appear to give you a better night's sleep, the quality of that sleep may not be as good as with natural sleep, and so you may not be any further ahead. And most sleep medications are psychologically addictive, if not physically addictive. The strategies discussed in Chapter 4 about good sleep to combat fatigue may help with cognitive adaptation as well. Good sleep hygiene and regular exercise can go a long way in helping you to sleep better and gain energy to do what you have to do in your day.

Joan listened to the advice the occupational thera-pist gave her. She tried to do some form of exercise at least three days a week. When Brent was home, they went for a walk in the evenings after dinner, and she re-ally enjoyed this time with him without the distraction of the TV or his computer. Once a week she went to a special class at the YMCA for breast cancer survivors. The atmosphere in the class was relaxed, and she felt at home with the other women who had been through similar experiences. They even joked about not remem-bering the exercises from one week to the next. This made her feel almost normal.

Lilly had also talked to her about changing the way she saw the substitute teacher's role in her classroom. That really helped her; she started to see her as a help instead of a replacement. Pat was a good teacher, and the kids really liked her. Joan was able to sit at her desk instead of getting up to help the kids, and she did a lot of one-on-one work with the weaker students. She found that she was able to concentrate on one student better than on the whole class. She even found herself thinking that this two-teacher approach was much bet-ter for the kids than if it were just her alone.

TAKE-HOME MESSAGES

Cognitive changes after treatment for cancer are very com-mon and very frightening for cancer survivors and their fam-ily. The changes often are subtle and may go unnoticed for a while as the survivor adapts to them and tries to function normally. These changes can have a significant effect on the person's ability to function both socially and in the workplace. It is important for survivors to report any changes to their healthcare provider so that appropriate referrals can be made to help them adjust to these changes and mitigate their effect.

CHAPTER 9

BEING A PART OF IT ALL

O f the estimated 12 million cancer survivors in the United States today, almost 40% are adults who were working at the time of diagnosis. Most of these will need to return to work after their treatment is over, and some may have worked through all or part of their treatment. Work is important, and for many, it is a necessity to support oneself and one's family. But work also provides us with self-esteem and validation of our role as men and women in the 21st century. It provides opportunities for social contact, intellectual stimulation, and personal growth.

Going back to work has been linked with overall survival after cancer, and survivors who return to work report feeling better. Going back to work after treatment for cancer is also a symbolic transition from the world of being a patient to the world of normality.

But being diagnosed with cancer can also change one's priorities in life. Some people discover that they don't want to keep working in the same job; the cancer may prompt them to do something different, make a change, or retire and focus on family and things that make them feel good rather than the daily grind.

Ben is a commodities trader, a bright, young over-achiever in a high-stress world of big money and bigger risk. At 25 years old, he works 60–70 hours a week and often goes to a bar or restaurant with his colleagues from work. His world came crashing down last year when his ankle broke during a late-night basketball game with his friends. He did not expect to hear what the emergency department doctor told him as he lay on a stretcher:

"It's cancer, I'm afraid, bone cancer. You're going to need to stay here for a while."

The rest was a blur. He had chemotherapy first, and then they amputated his leg below the knee. He went to a rehab hospital for three weeks. Then they sent him home with crutches and an appointment to see someone to make a prosthetic leg for him. For days he didn't answer his phone and didn't check his e-mail. His parents were frantic, and after three days of no contact, his mother arrived from Montana. She forced him to eat and drink, just a little bit every hour, and made sure that he bathed. She stayed for six weeks but then had to return to work and her husband.

"And what about your work?" she asked him one morning.

WHY GO BACK TO WORK?

Besides the loftier reasons to work as described earlier, most people have to work not only for the money but also for health insurance. Other survivors are eager to get back to work, especially if the work inspires them and makes them feel worthwhile. Still others have no choice and have to go back to work, perhaps even before they feel ready and healthy enough.

Variation exists in return-to-work statistics based on the type of cancer and the treatments given. Survivors with certain kinds of cancer appear to have greater success in returning to work; those with breast, prostate, and testicular cancer have relatively high rates of return. Others, such as those with brain, colorectal, lung, and head and neck cancers, have lower rates of return to the workforce; these cancers may carry higher rates of disability and a slower or more complicated recovery. It is well established that brain cancer survivors experience more limitations in their ability to work because of challenges with cognitive, psychological, and social functioning as a result of the cancer and its treatments.

Most cancer survivors have gone back to work one year after diagnosis (estimated to be about 60%–70%), and most stay for five to seven years. Of those who retire, about half say that it is unrelated to the cancer. In a study of adults with cancer, about half had changed some aspect of their jobs or worked less, but again reported that this had nothing to do with the cancer.

Ben had not thought much about work over the past weeks. Because he had not checked his e-mail, he was not sure what was happening there, and he didn't know who had tried to contact him. The battery for his cell phone had died long ago, so he didn't even know which of his colleagues had tried to call him. And his boss? What must he think? Ben had left a drugged message on his voice mail the morning he started chemotherapy and had not contacted him since.

But how could he face them all? He hadn't worn anything other than shorts since he got home from rehab. He wondered briefly how weird his pants would look with one leg half-empty and flapping around. He hadn't bothered contacting the place where they could make him a prosthetic leg, and the thought of using crutches in the office was daunting.

However, his mother was relentless. He knew how badly she needed to go back to his dad and her life in Montana, but she refused to even book a flight until he had at least talked to his boss. With a dry mouth and a fluttering heart, he called him on a Monday morning.

"Ben! We've been concerned about you! HR has been trying to reach you for weeks. Did you fall off the face of the earth? Are you okay?"

The normally cool-as-a-cucumber Ronald Brigham sounded flustered and unsure of what to say.

"Um, yeah, I guess I'm okay. I, um, well, I think I should maybe be thinking about coming back . . . if there's still a place for me."

"Of course there is! But you need to talk to HR. They know the rules and all that. How about you give them a call?"

Ben wrote down the number with a shaking hand. What was he so scared about?

WHAT MAKES GOING BACK TO WORK EASIER?

A number of factors can influence how well reintegration into the workforce goes. The first is the willingness of the organization or workplace to make accommodations for the cancer survivor, especially around flexible work hours and assignments, clearly identified support in the workplace, and a positive attitude on the part of coworkers. Respect for the changing needs of the cancer survivor is also noted as an important factor in successful return to work. For some survivors, a gradual return-to-work schedule will help to reduce stress and allow for rest and attendance at rehab and other medical appointments without the employee being perceived as missing work again or being absent repeatedly. Disclosing some information about the cancer to coworkers also has been reported to result in more positive responses from them. However, how much is disclosed is at the discretion of the survivor, and no one else (supervisor or HR staff) should do this on the person's behalf, especially without permission.

Some types of work also allow for more flexibility in work hours and duties. Those in so-called white-collar jobs appear to experience fewer challenges in the workplace than those whose jobs involve manual labor. Studies have found that younger men and those with advanced education and higher-level positions have an easier time returning and adjusting to work. This may reflect greater commitment to the work and more accommodation of the worker than in lower paying and less prestigious jobs.

Larger organizations also may provide more structure and guidance for reintegrating workers and may have policies in place. However, a study of medium to large companies found that half of the employers did not know the number of employees with a history of cancer, and only 38% had written guidelines to support policy in this area.

Ben met with Kathy, one of the staff from HR. She was about his age and he found the whole meeting very uncomfortable. He'd only seen her once before, at the office holiday party the year he started at the company, and he dimly remembered that they had flirted briefly while waiting for drinks at the bar. And now she was going to decide how he was going to do his work.

The whole day had not gone well. Earlier he couldn't find anything that fit; he knew he'd lost weight, but he was shocked at how much. His pants had slipped down and rested on his hip bones, and he had to rummage in his closet to find a belt to hold them up. The belt notches told the rest of the story—three inches past where he last buckled. And he was not sure what to do about the empty pant leg. His mom suggested just leaving it as is, but he tried to pin it below his knee and that just depressed him so much that he couldn't even look at it. He left it flapping. His shirt hung on his shoulders and his neck stuck out like a feathered chicken.

Kathy chattered away for most of the meeting. She didn't make eye contact, and he was almost glad for that. She asked questions, and he answered as best he could, mostly "yes" and "no" and "I think so." At the end he could hardly remember what the questions were. As he stood up to leave, forgetting for an instant that he needed to use his crutches and nearly falling over, she put out her hand to shake his, but his hands were on the crutches and she blushed, and they were done. As he waited for the taxi, all he could remember was that he had agreed to come back on Monday, back into his old job and those 70-hour weeks. What had he done?

WHAT ARE THE PITFALLS TO LOOK OUT FOR?

Cancer survivors are more than 50% more likely to be unemployed than their healthy counterparts. The treatment takes its toll physically and mentally, and some survivors may not be able to go back into their old jobs and may not be able to find new employment. Being off for long periods without wage protection places cancer survivors and their families in great financial jeopardy, so some may take jobs that are not suitable or are outside of their area of expertise or liking, just to earn a wage.

Going back to work too early may threaten survivors' ability to succeed at work. Having to take time off for medical appointments and to rest may make them vulnerable to criticism and the appearance of not pulling their weight, and perhaps even dismissal. About 20% of cancer survivors report limitations in what they are able to do at work, especially in the first five years after diagnosis.

While some impairments may be more obvious (amputation, for example), others are not visible and yet significantly affect the cancer survivor's return to work. Fatigue, cognitive changes, depression, and chronic pain are examples of invisible factors that affect work performance. Cognitive changes appear to pose the most difficulty, along with work that requires physical strength and stamina. Cancer survivors may also not do well in jobs that require deep concentration for long periods and keeping pace with learning new tasks and skills. Other factors that affect success include problems with coworkers and changes to duties and responsibilities that are outside of what the survivor can manage.

Cancer survivors who feel that they are supported by their employer and whose needs are accommodated do much better than those who have a negative experience when returning to work. The attitude of coworkers and supervisors is important. In a study of more than 200 supervisors, 66% stated that they believed that cancer survivors would not be able to perform their jobs properly when they came back to work after treatment, and 27% of coworkers were worried that they would have to pick up the slack when the cancer survivor was not able to perform to the expected level.

Some personal factors influence success when going back to work as well. Being older with other illnesses in addition to the cancer, having less education, having a lower income, and working in physical labor all reduce the chances that going back to work will work out for the cancer survivor. Not liking one's job makes it even more difficult to go back after having treatment. If the person no longer wants to progress in the job and is not motivated to do well, it is much harder to have a good attitude. If the individual suffers from depression or anxiety, the return to work is likely to be more challenging. And if the survivor's health is poor and ongoing issues with treatment side effects like fatigue are present, the person is less likely to succeed at being back at work.

Ben didn't sleep much in the nights before he went back to work. His mom left on Saturday, and he spent most of Sunday lying in bed, trying to figure out how he was going to do his old job. He tried to think about what he did all day, but it felt like so long ago that he could barely remember anything other than the noise of the phones ringing and the background roar of the other hundred traders yelling over the noise. He could see the trading floor, the computer screens glowing with the changing graphs, but mostly he saw the other traders, all of them standing at their desks or rushing to get a drink and then piling into taxis to go out for a late dinner or to play basketball. He could do NONE of that—not the standing nor the moving freely or playing basketball. He had a sinking feeling in his stomach that this was not going to go well.

He got to work early on Monday morning. He didn't want the trading floor to be full of people when he came in on his crutches, so he thought that if he got there really early, they would not stare at him as he made his way to his desk. It was almost empty when he got there, and he managed to get to his seat without attracting much attention. His colleagues showed up soon after he did. For the most part, they came over and greeted him with cautious slaps on the back and wary eyes.

"Hey, pal, good to see you! Drink after work, okay?"

"Hi, Ben! How ya doing? Long time no see."

But they were careful around him, and every now and then he caught one of them staring at him and the crutches that lay on the floor under his desk.

His boss didn't come to see him that first day, or the second, and by the third day, Ben felt so uncomfortable that he couldn't figure out what to do about it. Just before he left on Friday evening, exhausted and feeling like a wet noodle, he saw his boss standing in the entrance way to the trading floor.

"Hey, Ben, a word, if you please. In my office. Now. Okay?"

His exhaustion was replaced by nausea and dread. What did the boss want?

WHEN THINGS GO BAD

Unfortunately, discrimination in the workplace is still alive and well, and cancer survivors are sometimes the recipients of that discrimination. Cancer survivors have made legal claims against employers because of dismissal without cause, layoffs, wage issues, and demotions. The survivors often are more successful in winning their claims than other workers who file grievances, which provides evidence that cancer survivors do in fact face discrimination and different treatment. These issues tend to be worse for workers who have to do physical labor. However, cancer survivors tend to be hired less often into positions that demand physical labor. Claims under the Americans with Disabilities Act are more likely to be about interpersonal issues at work. The number of cancer survivors who file claims is relatively small, but it is a sign that discrimination in the workplace occurs.

Discrimination in the workplace may be overt or hidden. *Overt discrimination* can occur by means of slurs, threatening words or actions on the part of coworkers or supervisors, or other hostile acts. The environment itself may be hostile with lack of accommodation for someone with a disability. *Covert discrimination* most often presents as being passed over for promotion or denied benefits. All of this violates the Americans with Disabilities Act, which covers cancer survivors because cancer is regarded as a disease that affects or impairs a major life activity, work. Not all workers are covered under this act, and claims are decided on a case-by-case basis. Under this act, if an employer has more than 15 employees, reasonable accommodation must be made for workers with a disability as long as this does not pose an undue hardship on the business. This means that the employer does not have to make any changes that would be difficult or cost a lot of money, taking into consideration the size of the company and its resources. The employer also does not have to supply the worker with aids to help the person do the job better and is not expected to make allowances for lower-quality output from the worker. Under this act, the employer cannot use the disability as the basis for firing an employee, denying benefits, or refusing to hire someone. In terms of employees with cancer, the employer must make reasonable accommodations in work hours and allowing time off for medical appointments.

Another law, the Family and Medical Leave Act (FMLA), applies to companies with more than 50 employees. This act requires that all employees are allowed to take up to 12 weeks of unpaid leave in any 12-month period for medical purposes or to take care of a sick child or other family member with a serious health condition. During this time, the employer must continue to provide health insurance and other benefits. FMLA also allows for reduced work schedules when medically necessary. The act states that when employees return to work, they must be placed in the same or an equivalent position to the one they held before taking their medical leave.

Ben's boss was not alone. Kathy from HR was there as well, and Ben stumbled on his crutches as he moved onto the lush carpet.

"Sit down, please, Ben," began Kathy. "You've been back, what, a week, right?"

Ben nodded; his voice seemed to have left him.

"I, we, wanted to talk to you about how things were going," Kathy continued.

"Let's cut to the chase here, Kathy," Ronald said. "I'm going to level with you, Ben. A couple of the guys have talked to me about you."

"What do you mean? What did they say?" Ben was trying hard to think, but the thumping of his heart made the words jumble.

"Well, mostly stuff about you not carrying your weight. Nonsense mostly. I told them that I trust you and that they should keep their opinions to themselves. The cancer was in your leg, right? Not your brain. My dad is a Vietnam vet, and he came back without one arm. Never stopped him from doing anything, but they sure tried at times. You just do your best. Not any better than the guys, but not any worse. Okay?"

Ben saw the struggle in his jaw as he tried to control his emotions. So his dad was an amputee? Interesting. But then Kathy interrupted.

"Maybe we should talk more about what your needs are on the trading floor. Let's make an appointment for next week, and we can see if we need to change anything to make things easier for you."

MAKING GOING BACK TO WORK, WORK

Cancer survivors are often told by their healthcare providers that they can return to work when they "feel ready," but this is a vague statement. "Feeling ready" may not mean being able to go back, just that you want or need to go back. Although it is important to ask your healthcare provider about going back to work, consulting someone who specializes in back-to-work issues, particularly for the kind of work you do, may be a good idea. An occupational health specialist can be of great help. Your company or health insurance may know a specialist to refer you to. The occupational health specialist will assess your physical and emotional readiness to return to your specific job, the work environment, and other factors that may affect your ability to be successful once again.

It's important to make plans about going back to work while you are still away on leave. There may be a cancer rehabilitation program affiliated with the hospital or cancer center where you were treated. The specialists there may provide you with valuable support and strategies for maximizing your strength and resilience. Studies have shown that a combination of physical, vocational, and psychological rehabilitation is helpful for cancer survivors *before* they return to work.

Working with the occupational health specialist, you can develop a written plan that you should share with your supervisor and even your coworkers if appropriate. The plan should outline how many hours you can work, the type of work you can do, how your hours will increase over time if your return to work is graduated, and the date when you will be able to fulfill the duties of the position without accommodations. You should go over the plan with your supervisor regularly and make changes as required. If you cannot meet the requirements of the plan, you may need further rehabilitation, and the plan may need to be revised with a different end date or modified work responsibilities. Sharing this plan with your coworkers may help avoid the perception that you are getting special treatment or being allowed to slack off.

> *The first few weeks were hard for Ben. He felt as if a hundred pairs of eyes were boring into his back. He tried to show no signs of weakness and had found a way to stand at his desk like all the others, but he had to lean against it to maintain his balance. At the end of the day his back and leg were in great pain, but at least he looked like all the other traders, standing on the floor and yelling into the phone. And he had made an appointment to see the guy about the prosthetic leg. Ben hated the crutches, and without them he could maybe pass for normal. And maybe then he could go back to the gym and do some work to bulk up a bit and not look so scary. His mom and dad were so proud of*

*him when he told them that. He could hear the tears in
his mom's voice, but this time they were happy tears.
Or something like that.*

TAKE-HOME MESSAGES

Returning to work is a necessity for many cancer survivors for financial reasons, but working is also good for self-esteem and feelings of self-worth. The process can be difficult for some, and ongoing problems with fatigue and cognition present special challenges. Although laws exist to protect workers from discrimination in the workforce, subtle and outright discrimination does occur. Furthermore, cancer survivors sometimes have problems with coworkers who perceive that the survivor will no longer be able to do his or her job. A consultation with an occupational health specialist and a comprehensive plan can go far in anticipating and avoiding problems when the survivor returns to his or her place of employment.

CHAPTER 10

UP CLOSE AND PERSONAL

S exuality is much more than what we do in bed (or in the kitchen or on the living room floor!). How we see ourselves as men and women is an integral part of who we are as sexual beings. So, too, is who we are attracted to, physically and emotionally. Our sexuality is part of self-expression, self-image, and self-esteem. It is sometimes said that sex itself (the act) is the glue that holds couples together, and without that glue, couples start to drift apart until they live like college roommates—friendly yet not intimate.

Sex is often the last thing on a person's mind when in the middle of treatment and not feeling well. But eventually the idea pops up again, and couples often are surprised when it does. This also is often the time when difficulties that previously were not there become apparent. Sexual difficulties can happen to anyone, at any age, and with any kind of cancer diagnosis. Many people may think that problems only occur in survivors who have cancer in organs directly related to sexual functioning (prostate, uterus or cervix, breast). However, up to 80% of cancer survivors experience some degree of difficulty with their sexuality after treatment. But not all of them want to talk about it or do anything about it. Many couples say that the cancer drew them closer than they ever were before, but that intensity often fades over time, and people want to go back to the way things were before.

> *Eric is 62 years old. Shortly after he retired from the bank where he had worked for 35 years, he was diagnosed with prostate cancer. What bad timing! He had so many plans for his retirement, including working on a sailboat with his brother who lived in Florida, and all his plans were ruined. His wife, Jo, tried to placate him, telling him it was just a bump in the road, but ever since the surgery to remove his prostate, he has been depressed and grumpy. Jo has been walking on eggshells around him. The surgery was almost 18 months ago, and he was now a different person. He seemed to have lost his zest for life. She wasn't sure how she could reach him. Things were different between them too—he didn't touch her anymore, and on the one or two occasions when she tried to initiate sex, he had rebuffed her and slept on the couch those nights. What was she going to do?*

WHAT ARE THE MOST COMMON SEXUAL PROBLEMS AFTER TREATMENT?

Sexual problems that occur after cancer can be grouped into the following categories:
- Body image changes
- Changes in the desire for sex

- Arousal difficulties
- Problems with orgasm
- Pain
- Hormonal changes.

Men and women will experience these challenges slightly differently because of the differences in their sexual organs and also because of how they have been socialized to see and experience themselves as sexual beings.

Body image is a central aspect of how we see ourselves as sexual beings. Women appear to have poorer body image than men, in part because women have traditionally received very clear and pervasive messages about what they are supposed to look like and dress like and what is seen as "sexy" by the media, a constantly changing target. But men are not immune to similar messages, and changes to their bodies after cancer also may bring about feelings of vulnerability and fears that they are not sexually attractive to their partner. The most common changes that interfere with sexual self-image include surgical scars, such as mastectomy, amputations, and ostomies (a passage from the abdomen to the outside to get rid of waste products), weight gain or loss, lymphedema (swelling of a limb or body part due to blockages or removal of lymph nodes), and shrinkage of the male genitalia. In men with prostate cancer who are prescribed androgen deprivation therapy (ADT) to lower testosterone levels, the medication causes weight gain, loss of muscle mass, and breast enlargement. Men with these symptoms often describe feeling sexually unattractive.

Women who have had a mastectomy commonly report challenges with accepting their new bodies after the surgery. Even if they have had reconstruction, the new breast may not look

or feel the way their "old" breast used to, and the reconstruct-
ed breast is a symbol of the cancer and all that it represents.

Sexual desire or libido is another facet of sexuality that is frequently affected by the cancer, its treatment, or other long-term
effects of treatment, such as fatigue. Despite some erroneous
beliefs about men's sexual desire always being stronger or higher than women's, both men and women frequently experience
a loss of desire with the shock of diagnosis that commonly persists through treatment. However, some couples find that their
desire for sex and the intimate connection resulting from sexual touch drives their desire higher in the days after diagnosis.

Other reasons cause people to lose their desire for sexual activity. Pain or the medications used to treat pain (usually opi-
oids) can lower desire. Fatigue is another primary cause of lack
of desire. If the partner of a survivor believes that sexual activity is causing the survivor discomfort or pain, or the survivor
does not seem to be enjoying the activity, this in turn can lower desire for the partner. It's complicated!

Changes in arousal, or the inability to become aroused, are
very common sexual side effects of cancer treatment. Men who
have had surgery to remove the prostate gland frequently lose
their ability to have an erection. This can occur in up to 100%
of men. Recovery from this depends in part on the skill of the
surgeon in preventing damage to the fragile nerves responsible for erection, what the man's erections were like before the
surgery, and whether aggressive postoperative penile rehabilitation is suggested and complied with. Surgery anywhere in the
pelvis, for example, for colon cancer, can have similar effects.

The equivalent arousal response in women is related to
vaginal lubrication. Many drugs can affect this in women.

Anything that shuts down ovarian function and production of estrogen will cause a decrease in lubrication and vaginal dryness. This can be painful and can result in an avoidance of sexual activity, as well as a responsive lack of desire on the part of the woman.

Changes in the **ability to have an orgasm** can lead to lack of satisfaction with sexual activity. For some, this can cause relationship problems. This may be caused by physical changes as a result of surgery or emotional issues related to the cancer, fear of recurrence, or fear of pain. Men who have had their prostate removed often complain that orgasm is not as pleasurable or intense as it was before. However, some men report that their orgasms are *more* intense, almost painful, after the surgery.

In women, surgical removal of the uterus and cervix may result in changes in the sensation of orgasm. The uterus is known to contract during orgasm, and so absence of the organ itself may be responsible. However, this change also may be due to the destruction of key nerves during surgery.

Sexual pain is a common side effect after surgery to sexual organs and, as mentioned earlier, can be a result of hormonal changes.

Hormonal changes may occur after chemotherapy, radiation therapy, or surgery. It is well accepted that men's desire is driven by testosterone, and so when this hormone is lowered by ADT for the treatment of advanced prostate cancer, one of the first things the man may notice is that his libido disappears. This happens to about 85% of men on ADT. Men describe life with no testosterone as being devoid of an essential part of themselves. They don't think of sex, don't want sex, and don't notice an attractive person, including their partner.

They also stop touching their partner, not even a hug or a kiss on the cheek. This lack of touch can be extremely distressing for the partner.

Radiation to the head may affect the pituitary gland and result in altered hormone levels, which can result in profound changes in sexual desire. For example, if the pituitary gland produces too much of a hormone called *prolactin,* this will drive down a man's testosterone level, reducing his sexual desire.

Many women with hormone receptor–positive breast cancer are prescribed medication for years after their primary treatment to reduce the risk of recurrence. These drugs (selective estrogen receptor modulators and aromatase inhibitors) drastically reduce levels of estrogen in the body and lead to vaginal dryness, pain with penetration, and lack of libido.

Any and all of these can lead to significant changes to a couple's sex life—and to how they see themselves as individuals in the relationship. Some couples are quite happy in a sexless relationship, but this is not always the case. To go back to the glue analogy, a relationship with no physical touching can lead to emotional distancing. Some couples argue, whereas others avoid the whole situation and just drift apart.

> *Jo didn't know what to do about Eric. He was obviously suffering and unhappy, and yet he would not talk to her. This was not unusual for him; he was one of those "silent" types who had a hard time expressing emotions. It had caused them problems early in their marriage, but they compromised, and over time she got used to his silences and didn't take them per-*

sonally. But this she was taking personally. He didn't touch her anymore: not a good-bye kiss when he went to meet his buddies for coffee, no hand-holding when they went to the movies, nothing. He was also much more secretive about things, too. He never undressed in front of her anymore, and he locked the bathroom door when he was in there. She hadn't really paid that much attention to these changes, but as she thought about it, she realized that all this had started about two weeks after he came home from the hospital.

She talked to her friend Ruth about this, swearing her to secrecy. Ruth's husband, Bill, had also been diagnosed with prostate cancer. Even though he'd had radiation treatment, Jo thought that Ruth might be able to help. They talked one day when they went for a walk around the golf course. Was that ever enlightening! Ruth told her that some men have problems with leakage of urine after their surgery that lasts for months or even years. And then there was the sex part—Ruth said that Bill had been having problems in that department, so he went to his doctor and had all sorts of pills to try. Jo listened, partly fascinated and partly horrified. How did Ruth know all of this? She couldn't wait to get home and ask Eric about this. But how was she going to do that?

TALKING ABOUT IT

It can be really difficult to talk about sensitive issues like sexuality and feelings, even with the person who is closest to us. For many couples, sex has just happened over the years, and there has been no need to talk about it. But when problems arise, you need to talk. Where do you start? Bringing up the topic can be fraught with tension, and emotions can run high. But the longer you leave it, the harder it will be to have the conversation. Days turn to weeks, and before you know it, months have gone by and the lack of sex or touching becomes the 300-pound gorilla in the room—always present, often menacing, and hard to ignore.

- Start the conversation by stating how the situation affects *you*. Use only "I" statements, and don't talk about what you think the other person is feeling. Own your own feelings and the effect that this is having on *you*.

- Take turns talking, and really **listen** to what your partner is saying. We often don't listen well—we are so busy thinking of our response to what the other person is saying that we miss most of what they are trying to tell us.

- Don't interrupt or make assumptions about what the other person means. Seek clarification if you don't fully understand or if you are confused about something.

- Paraphrase what you have been told. "So you are saying that this is the way you have been feeling for the past six months?" is an example of paraphrasing.

- Consider getting some professional help if it is too difficult or painful to have a good discussion about what is going on. Resources for finding help will be provided in Chapter 12.

Jo asked Eric to go for a walk after dinner one night.
She was very nervous and had hardly eaten anything.

As soon as they left the path from their house, she took a deep breath.

"Honey? What's wrong? You seem so . . . different somehow. Is there something you're not telling me? Have you seen the doctor, is that it?"

Eric's voice was strained. "It's nothing, okay? It's my problem and I'll sort it out!"

Jo took another breath.

"No, Eric, it's not your problem! It's my problem because you are different and I'm worried, so that makes it my problem too! What is it? Are you having an affair? Is that it? Oh my goodness, that's it, isn't it? You're having an affair and you want to leave me."

Her voice rose in fear and Eric's response took her by surprise.

"An affair? Oh, Jo, you couldn't be further from the truth." And Eric laughed.

"Then tell me what's going on, Eric. Tell me!"

And Eric told her. He described the constant leaking of urine that he had been trying so hard to hide from her.

"Is that why you dress in the bathroom?" she asked, confusion flitting over her face.

Yes, he admitted. He was wearing diapers. He was keeping them hidden in the bathroom where she couldn't see them.

"And is that why you won't touch me? In case I feel them?"

Once again he admitted that he was avoiding her because he was afraid that one thing would lead to another, and he wouldn't be able to make love to her. His

erections were gone, completely gone. And he didn't
know what to do.
  And then he started to cry.

WHAT CAN HELP WITH SEXUAL PROBLEMS?

Avoidance can lead to all sorts of trouble. Avoidance often feels like personal rejection, and this hurts, a lot. When you don't talk about what is bothering you, your partner may make assumptions. Then the assumptions become the truth in the partner's eyes. It is far better to talk about it than to let assumptions simmer.

Some strategies can help in solving sexual problems after cancer. The first thing to do is to seek out information about what is happening and why. Asking your oncology care provider to explain why this is happening is the first step. Your oncologist or nurse can refer you to someone to talk to about communication problems in your relationship. There are social workers, psychologists, and therapists to do this part of the work. But ask your healthcare team if there are any physical reasons (for example, side effects from surgery) or treatment-related effects (such as from medication you are taking) that may be involved in the sexual challenges you are having.

It is always a good idea to take your partner with you to all your appointments. Four ears are better than two. Your partner can ask additional questions or seek clarification when you are trying to take in what is being talked about. Your partner can take notes, too, so that you have a written reminder of what was discussed. And this involves your partner too—it does take two to tango, after all!

Some specific strategies exist for finding solutions to the most common sexual problems encountered after treatment. They are, of course, dependent on the reason for the problem and whether treatment is available. Many survivors, like anyone else, look for quick fixes, a pill or potion that will fix whatever is wrong with minimal effort and involvement. Unfortunately, this does not work for sexual problems, which tend to be complex in origin and manifestation.

Problems with accepting a **new or altered body** are not that easy to solve. We all have an image in our heads of what we look like, and many of us judge our physical appearance harshly. This is an area where counseling can really help. Our partner usually does not see us as we see ourselves. They tend to love us, warts and all, and talking about the physical changes and what these mean can be helpful in accepting these changes. A counselor or marital/couples therapist can be very helpful in getting couples to talk to one another in a calm and productive atmosphere. The counselor can ask questions to help draw out issues that may be scary for you to talk about. The counselor helps to control the conversation and keeps it constructive. A skilled counselor can really help a couple get to the heart of the matter and help find solutions to the problems.

The counselor or therapist may suggest some homework for the couple to do. One very useful exercise to help people accept physical changes is something called *sensate focus exercises.* These exercises help cancer survivors to get in touch with their body as a source of pleasure instead of pain and suffering, as is so often the case after going through treatment. The exercises allow a couple to reconnect in a gradual and pleasurable way in their own time and at their own pace. Instructions on how to do these exercises are included in Chapter 12.

Problems with **sexual desire** are probably the hardest issue to solve. Sexual desire is a very fragile phenomenon, and there is no magic bullet (pill or potion) that can increase desire or bring it back when it is gone. Men seem to respond well to testosterone replacement if levels of this hormone are low. However, men who have had prostate cancer usually are advised to avoid supplemental testosterone because it is believed that this can cause the cancer to come back. Women without ovaries also appear to experience increased desire when given testosterone, but no approved form of testosterone therapy exists for women at the present time. There are also concerns that testosterone is broken down in the female body into estrogen, so its use in women with hormone receptor–positive breast cancer or other hormonally dependent cancer is not widely accepted. Studies of medication to increase libido in women have also shown a strong placebo effect. That means that in the women who took the sugar pill, increases in the anticipated effect were equal to those of the women who took the medication. This is an interesting finding; perhaps if a woman thinks that something is going to help, it will. So maybe medication is not the way to go in treating low libido, but rather talking about it will help just as much!

One strategy that does seem to help women (this has not been studied in men) is telling them that desire is not a necessary precursor to sexual activity. Many women find that once they are aroused, after some kissing and cuddling, their desire happens at that point. This is useful information to many women who love their partner and want to be sexual with them. If they wait for spontaneous desire, it might never happen, but if they start "fooling around," then responsive desire may occur.

Arousal problems are usually treated depending on the cause. In men with erectile difficulties, drugs such as sildenafil (Viagra®), tadalafil (Cialis®), and vardenafil (Levitra®) may help. These medications prevent blood from leaving the penis once physical stimulation has encouraged blood flow to the organ and are partially dependent on intact erectile nerves to maintain the erection. Not all men can take these medications. They cause a lowering of blood pressure, and men who take nitrates for chest pain should not take them. They have a number of side effects including headache, facial flushing, heartburn, back pain, and nasal congestion. They are also quite expensive and may not be covered by health insurance. More invasive strategies for getting and maintaining an erection include a penile pump and penile self-injection, in which a small amount of medication is injected into the side of the penis to cause it to fill with blood. Both of these methods require some physical dexterity, and some men are put off by the invasiveness of them, but they do work for some men and should be considered.

Arousal problems in women usually involve lack of vaginal lubrication as discussed previously. A number of strategies can help with this, and most are well accepted by women and their partners. The use of vaginal moisturizers can help counteract vaginal dryness for daily comfort. They are usually not sufficient for sexual activity but may help with mild dryness. Examples of vaginal moisturizers are Replens® and K-Y® Liquibeads™. They are used three to four times per week and are available over the counter at most drugstores in North America.

ca. Lubricants are used to improve and enhance comfort during sexual activity. There are a number of good lubricants readily available in drugstores, including water-based products (Astroglide®, FriXion™, and Embrace®). These may contain glycerin (check the ingredient list on the box), which some women find irritating. Many water-based lubricants are available that don't contain glycerin, including Liquid Silk™, Oh My™ (organic), Probe®, and Slippery Stuff®. These are only available through online retailers and at sex stores. Silicone-based lubricants are especially effective because they stay slippery for a long time. They need to be removed with soap and water if they spill on the skin. K-Y® Intrigue, Eros®, Wet Platinum®, and Pink® are other examples of silicone-based lubricants. Some women prefer to use natural oils (almond, olive, or coconut), but these will destroy latex condoms and if they remain in the vagina and are not flushed out, they can become rancid. Douching is not recommended for any women, as it destroys a woman's natural vaginal milieu, so ensuring that oils do not remain inside the body can pose a problem. For some women, the only effective treatment is local estrogen (in the form of a cream, ring, or pessary) in the vagina. This is a controversial topic among oncologists when treating women with hormone receptor–positive breast cancer.

Problems with **orgasm** are quite difficult to treat. The involvement of a certified sex therapist can be helpful in this regard. Many people are unsure of exactly what a sex therapist does. For a start, a sex therapist does NOT watch couples have sex and does NOT require any form of nudity in sessions. Most sex therapists in North America are certified by the American Association of Sexuality Educators, Counselors, and Therapists

(AASECT, www.aasect.org) and have years of education and supervision before becoming certified. The AASECT Web site
has a list of certified therapists in your area or close to you.
The therapist may, among other strategies, suggest the use of
vibrators to increase sensation, pelvic floor physiotherapy to
help with loss of internal muscle tone, or sensate focus exercises to help reconnect with your partner.

Sexual pain may need to be treated by a medical specialist
such as a gynecologist or urologist. A pelvic floor physiotherapist can also be very helpful because pain is often related to
the muscles of the pelvic floor. The pelvic floor physiotherapist
has the expertise to assess how these muscles are functioning
and can suggest exercises and other treatments to relax these
muscles and reduce pain. Sexual pain can be quite difficult to
treat, as it usually has a related component of anxiety; the person anticipates the pain and contracts the muscles of the pelvic floor in response.

Hormonal changes resulting in sexual problems pose a challenge in treatment options. Obviously if a man is given drugs
to eradicate testosterone in his body, he cannot take more testosterone! And women who are taking medications to reduce
the amount of estrogen in their bodies may not want to take
anything that can potentially raise their levels of this hormone.
It should be noted that the use of vaginal estrogen does NOT
increase levels in the bloodstream significantly or at all (this
depends on the type and dose of the medication prescribed).
Most survivors who experience sexual changes as a result of
hormonal changes learn to live with the consequences. This
can be difficult for their partners and for the relationship.
There are many nonsexual ways of showing affection and pas-

sion for one's partner; however, after a lifetime of doing things one way, it can be difficult to learn new ways of being a sexual being and maintaining sexual intimacy within the relationship. A skilled sex therapist or counselor can provide the couple with new ideas and strategies to help with this.

> *Eric agreed to see his nurse practitioner about what was happening. He was no longer scheduled to see the urologist who had performed the surgery, and he liked Steve, who practiced at a nearby clinic. At the last minute he tried to postpone the appointment, claiming he had a headache, but Jo would not go along with that, so he reluctantly went. Steve, a young man in his early 30s, was very matter-of-fact when Jo described what was going on. Eric was having a hard time looking up from where his hands were gripped tightly in his lap.*
>
> *"Okay, Eric, so what have you tried to do about any of this? Let's start with the urinary incontinence. This is not uncommon after prostate cancer surgery, but 18 months seems to be a long time to still have this much leakage. How many pads are you using a day? What about at night?"*
>
> *Eric answered in a soft voice; this was so embarrassing, but part of him was glad to have the opportunity to talk about it. Steve then asked about erections. Eric blushed and mumbled his way through his responses.*
>
> *"This is also not unusual after this type of surgery, but I would expect to see some signs of recovery by*

now. Do you remember what the surgeon said about nerve sparing? I can look through your notes to see if there is a mention of this in the urologist's letter to us."

Eric looked blankly at Steve. He couldn't remember talking to the urologist at all after the surgery. He had been pumped so full of drugs that his hospital stay was just a blur.

"Okay, here it is," Steve had rifled through the chart and had found the letter. "It says here that you should start a course of penile rehabilitation with low-dose Viagra as soon as the catheter comes out. Did you do that?"

Eric shook his head. He remembered the nurse at the urologist's office saying something about this to him, and she had given him a package with papers in it, but he had put that somewhere when he came home and forgotten about it.

Now what?

WHAT CAN GET IN THE WAY OF GETTING HELP?

This can be a very difficult area to seek and get help. Survivors often think, and are led to believe, that they should just be happy to be alive, that sex is a luxury, and something you may have to give up in exchange for life. But sex—and our sexuality—is a very important part of quality of life. Just because you have had cancer does not mean that your quality of life should remain less than it could be.

Even though your healthcare team is aware that the treatments cause sexual problems, they often don't talk about this for a variety of reasons. They may not be sure that you want to know about this and don't want to appear to be interfering in your private life. Your doctors and nurses are people, just like the rest of us, and may find it difficult to talk about this. They may be afraid of blushing or stammering or being unable to answer any questions you may ask. You would be surprised to learn how little information about sexuality is taught in medical and nursing schools across the country. You may need to open the door to this discussion, and you will find that most will be willing to talk about it with you. But someone has to start the conversation!

You also don't have to do anything you don't want to. However, getting accurate information about the causes of sexual problems after treatment and learning what may help is a worthwhile first step in deciding what, if anything, you want to do about it. Some couples are content to leave things as they are. They may not even miss sexual activity and focus instead on a loving but not physical relationship. That is fine as long as it meets the needs of both individuals.

The life-altering experience of cancer also may precipitate the breakup of some relationships. In the aftermath of the diagnosis and the natural reevaluating of life that comes with that, some survivors may find that they no longer want to be in a relationship that does not meet their needs, whether physical, emotional, or spiritual, and choose to move forward without their spouse or partner. And in some instances the spouse or partner ends the relationship because they can't or don't want to continue in a relationship that may ask more of them than they are prepared to give.

WHAT IF YOU'RE SINGLE?

Sex and the single person after cancer is a topic that is not often addressed by healthcare providers. There is somehow an assumption that if you are not in a relationship, then you are not sexual. Nothing could be further from the truth. First, each of us is a sexual being in ourselves, and many single people have active sexual lives. Cancer survivors with erectile problems after treatment may still want to masturbate, and the lack of erections or ejaculate after prostate cancer surgery may come as a surprise. Women, too, will want to experience orgasms through masturbation, and altered sensations may be bothersome. Of course, partnered survivors may also masturbate; this is not something that only single people do!

What about telling a potential partner about the cancer? When do you tell? How much do you tell? There is no right or wrong answer to this. It all depends on the nature of the relationship and how you wish to see the relationship develop. Telling someone that you have had cancer on a first date may be premature; who knows if there is going to be a second date? But waiting too long (months or longer) may feel to the other person like you are hiding something. Some survivors wait to tell because they don't want to rehash the details of their treatment over again and deal with the perhaps emotional response of the other person, when the survivor has moved on and left those emotions behind. You may need to figure out a short and snappy way of telling someone that you have had cancer and then change the subject to avoid this, or you may need to be prepared to give the details and help the other person realize what living after cancer is all about. The choice is yours.

Steve, the nurse practitioner, gave Eric some medication samples to try at home. He carefully explained how they should be used, and Jo was a little upset when he told Eric to try them without her the first couple of times. Steve noticed the look on Jo's face.

"Don't worry, Jo. There's a reason for this. Often men are so anxious to be with their partner that they get performance anxiety, and even with the medication, they can't have an erection. I see this quite often. I've found that encouraging them to try the first couple of pills alone can help to reduce the anxiety, and then the pills really do work."

"Okay, I'll take your word for it. As long as at some point I can get involved . . ."

As the words left her mouth, Jo felt herself go red. She looked up at Eric and he had a smile on his face, a real smile, and she realized that it had been a long time since she had seen him smile like that.

"Come on, honey," she said as she stood up. "Let's get you home and doing your homework."

TAKE-HOME MESSAGES

Sexual difficulties are very common after cancer treatment. Many survivors suffer in silence and don't ask for help. Cancer treatment affects sexuality for different reasons, including changes in body image, surgery that affects normal sexual functioning, and chemotherapy and radiation therapy that affect sexual response. Help is available, and oncology care providers can refer survivors and their partner to specialized therapists who can provide suggestions for improving this important aspect of quality of life.

EMPTY NESTS

F ertility is very much a survivorship issue and most often becomes important some time after treatment is over. Unfortunately, it is also an issue that should have been addressed before treatment started, and not much can be done when treatment is over. The three most common modes of treatment for cancer—chemotherapy, radiation, and surgery—can all affect potential fertility. Surgery to the reproductive organs (uterus, cervix, ovaries, and testicles) may physically alter the survivor's ability to either conceive or, in the case of women, carry a fetus during pregnancy. Chemotherapy, because it interferes with cell growth, can temporarily or permanently shut down the ovaries or testicles and prevent eggs from ripening or sperm from being produced. Radiation can do the same, as well as cause structural damage to the testicles. Not being able to have children can be a devastating side effect of cancer with little hope for resolution.

> *Brad was diagnosed with testicular cancer when he was 15 years old. It was the scariest and the most embarrassing thing that had ever happened to him. His mom cried most of the time, and his dad took him to*

appointments. His dad was not one to show much emotion, and Brad never saw him upset through everything—the surgery and then the chemo. So Brad didn't show any emotion either, well, not to anyone else, but when he was alone, which was not that often, he bit the inside of his cheeks till they bled. He wasn't sure how his friends would be with him afterward, and going back to school with sprouts of hair like a chicken was the worst. But he got through it, and his friends were okay, better than okay, really. Now, at age 25, those days are ancient history . . . kind of. He has a prosthetic testicle where his own one was removed. Over the years he's gotten used to the feel of it, and his "guys" are a little lopsided. But the rest of the stuff works! And now he has met Brit, and they are getting married next summer. He's not sure what to tell her about his cancer. In fact, he's not sure himself what difference the cancer may mean to them.

HOW DOES CANCER AFFECT MALE FERTILITY?

Chemotherapy, surgery, and radiation can all affect male fertility. This may happen in one of two ways: The first is damage to the brain from radiation or chemotherapy that affects the production of hormones responsible for the development of mature sperm in the testicles. The second is from damage to the testicles from radiation given directly to the testicles or to the pelvic area. However, sperm are constantly being produced. If the cells that produce sperm recover (called *Leydig cells*), fertility may be preserved, but the man may produce fewer sperm or ones that are not as healthy as in an unaffected man.

HOW DOES CANCER AFFECT FEMALE FERTILITY?

Fertility in women, as it is in men, is controlled by hormones produced in response to signals from the brain. This causes the release of an egg (ovum) every month. Unlike men, who continually produce sperm, women are born with a finite number of eggs in the ovaries.

A woman also needs a functioning uterus to carry a pregnancy. Surgery to remove the uterus, ovaries, or cervix will result in an inability to conceive. Radiation to the pelvis can cause the ovaries to shrink and stop maturing eggs. Radiation to the uterus can cause structural damage that would prevent a pregnancy from continuing because the uterus could not increase in size as the fetus grows. Chemotherapy can cause the ovaries to stop producing hormones that cause ripening of the eggs on a monthly basis.

Most women do not have their normal menstrual cycle if their ovaries are damaged. This may be permanent, or their periods may come back months or years after treatment is over. Even if the menstrual cycle does start again, many women find that they have difficulties conceiving or they have early menopause, after which they cannot conceive. The older the woman is at the time of treatment, the less likely she is to recover her fertility.

Brad had been thinking about the cancer a lot since he proposed to Brit. He knew that they needed to talk about it, but he wasn't sure how to start the conversation. He asked his dad what he should do, but his dad told him to let bygones be bygones and to let the past stay where it was, behind him. That didn't feel right to Brad. So one sunny Saturday morning, he asked her to come over and he'd make her breakfast.

"Brit, honey, there's something you need to know."

Brit's face lost all color and tears sprang to her eyes.

"Honey, hang on, it's not bad. Well, not really. Oh man, how do I talk about this? This is embarrassing . . ."

"Just tell me, Brad. Just say it! If you want to break up, if you don't want to marry me—"

"No! Honey, it's so not that. I just . . . it's . . . oh, dammit—I had cancer. Like 10 years ago. That's all."

Brit took a breath and stared at him.

"Cancer? Where? How? How come you're only telling me now?"

Brad took a deep breath. "Well, my testicle. When I was fifteen. I thought you would have figured it out, you know, that I have a fake one."

Brit blushed, and it was now Brad's turn to be shocked. How could she not have known?

TALKING ABOUT FERTILITY AFTER CANCER

Like any sensitive topic, it can be really difficult to talk about this. If you had cancer as a child or teenager, your parents may not have talked to you about this, or only in vague terms, and they may not have been fully informed by your healthcare team at the time of your diagnosis. Or, in the chaos of learning that their child has cancer, many parents don't even think about what might happen 10, 20, or more years in the future. They just want their precious child to live at any cost, and considerations about something so far away are just not something they can even think about.

In adults newly diagnosed with cancer where treatment may affect fertility, the amount of information they are given about this varies considerably. In the rush to start treatment, a discussion about the impact of the treatment on fertility may not occur. In a study of oncologists across the United States, 30% stated that their focus is on planning treatment and curing the cancer and not on the desires for childbearing in women with cancer. In another study, fewer than 50% of oncologists routinely referred their female patients to fertility specialists prior to treatment. In another study, 91% of oncology care providers felt that sperm banking should be offered to all male patients after puberty, but almost half of them also reported that they never bring up the topic with their male patients!

Among patients with cancer, the desire to one day have children is strong. Having a child is in some ways the opposite of having cancer; cancer is about fear and loss, whereas having children is about hope and life. When asked, more than 80% of female adolescent patients were interested in fertility preservation, but only 30% were willing to delay the start of treatment to preserve fertility. In men with cancer, just over 50% in one study had been told about sperm banking, but only 24% actually banked their sperm. Lack of information was cited as the reason they did not bank their sperm.

WHAT FERTILITY PRESERVATION OPTIONS ARE THERE?

The best options to preserve fertility currently exist for men and must happen before treatment begins. Sperm banking, in which semen is collected and then frozen at very low temperature, is an effective method for future conception; however, success is age dependent. For young men who have gone through puberty, masturbation to produce ejaculate that can be frozen is easy and does not require a significant delay to the start of treatment. Men can make more than one deposit but need to have a 48-hour window between samples. Younger teenagers may find this embarrassing, and it can be a difficult decision to make. Having to think about future fertility at a time when fatherhood is a distant and unreal concept can be really hard. Pressure from parents and care providers may further complicate matters. It costs money to bank sperm, and there is usually an annual fee to keep the sperm frozen, which may also be a barrier for some families.

Teenage patients with cancer who want to bank sperm may have some physical challenges to doing so. These mostly relate to embarrassment at having to masturbate and knowing that their parents know this too. Some teens may never have masturbated and may need some sensitive coaching. If the teen is unable to provide a sample in the lab, an alternative may be to do the collection at home and then take it to the lab, as long as the sample is kept at body temperature (place in a pocket against the chest) and delivered within an hour of collection. Kits that contain a cryopreservative to freeze the sample can be obtained and then mailed by express mail to the sperm bank. These kits are available through Fertile Hope (see Chapter 12), who may also be able to provide some financial support to families for fertility preservation.

The options for women are limited and must be acted upon before treatment starts. The option with the greatest likelihood of a successful pregnancy in the long term is the creation of an embryo that can be frozen. This has resulted in a successful pregnancy rate of about 50%. In order for this to happen, the woman must have a male partner and she must be able to wait at least one menstrual cycle before starting her cancer treatment. She has to undergo stimulation of the ovaries to produce multiple eggs, which are then mixed with her partner's sperm in a petri dish to create any number of embryos that are frozen and can be implanted into her uterus in the future. This whole process is expensive and requires the woman to delay treatment until the eggs have been harvested from her ovaries. If she is unable to carry a fetus, the embryos could also be implanted in the future into a surrogate, another woman who would carry the pregnancy and then give the baby to the couple. Women with hormone-dependent cancers cannot do this because of the high doses of hormones that have to be taken to stimulate the ovaries to produce multiple eggs. Freezing eggs or ovarian tissue is an experimental treatment at the present time; only 700 successful pregnancies have been reported worldwide using egg freezing.

For men and women who must have radiation to the pelvic area to treat cancer, it is common for the treating physician to try to protect the ovaries and testicles from direct radiation. This is done by using shields during radiation treatment, and in the case of some women, surgically moving the ovaries away from the treatment field and then putting them back in their usual place when treatment is over. However, radiation damage to the uterus may shrink it and make it less elastic, making carrying a pregnancy impossible.

> *Brad and Brit spent hours talking and a lot of that time crying. At first Brit was really upset that he hadn't told her the details of his cancer sooner. But then she realized that he couldn't remember the details of his treatment; he knew he had surgery and chemotherapy, but not the details of the drugs. And he really couldn't remember much of what the doctors had told him. Had they told him anything? He asked his dad about it, and once again his dad told him to let the past go.*
>
> *"I can't just let it go, Dad!" he shouted one day in frustration. "This impacts my future. Brit and I want to have kids, and if I can't have any, she needs to walk away now!"*
>
> *As the words left his mouth, the seriousness of what he said sunk in. Would she leave him if he couldn't have kids? He had to find out what the score was, and yet he was terrified that this could be the end of him and Brit. He had to find out more, and he had to do it quickly.*
>
> *He made an appointment to see his family doctor the following week. It had been 10 years since his can-*

cer diagnosis, and he no longer saw the doctors at the cancer clinic. Brit insisted on coming with him, and he was pleased that he did not have to do this alone.

Dr. Barnes was matter-of-fact, which helped a lot. Brad was so nervous that he could feel his heart beating in his chest like a bass drum. Brit had a notebook and wrote down every word. Dr. Barnes explained that it was pretty simple to check if he could father children—all that was needed was a semen sample that would be tested for the presence of sperm, their number, and how active they were. If all that was okay, they shouldn't have any problems. Brad could feel the relief flow over him like a warm shower.

WHAT DO PATIENTS WITH CANCER NEED TO KNOW ABOUT FERTILITY AFTER CANCER?

The provision of information about the effects of cancer treatment on future fertility is an area fraught with problems with recall and information overload. For the parents of a child or teenager with cancer, it may be just too much to take in while trying to cope with the diagnosis and treatment decisions. In one study, all the parents of male childhood patients with cancer were told about the impact of treatment on fertility, and yet only 50% of them recalled any information about this, and 36% denied receiving any information.

Various expert groups have published statements and guidelines, including the American Society for Reproductive Medicine and the American Society of Clinical Oncology (see Chap-

ter 12). However, not all physicians follow these recommendations and discuss fertility issues with their patients or the parents of their pediatric patients. In order to provide accurate information, these physicians need to keep up to date in a rapidly evolving field of medicine. Some may not be willing to do
so and may regard this as beyond their scope, which is to save
the lives of their patients with cancer, and leave these kinds of
issues to other experts when the cancer is cured. However, at a
minimum, they should refer their patients to a fertility expert,
preferably *before* treatment starts, as the impact on fertility may
influence their treatment decision. This usually does not happen because of the pressure to begin treatment, lack of fertility specialists in smaller towns and cities, and perception by the
patient or provider that this is not necessary at the time. When
consulting a fertility specialist, it is important to ensure that
the clinic and staff are fully accredited and not a fly-by-night
scheme with inadequate experience. The American Society for
Reproductive Medicine Web site (www.asrm.org) has information about qualified experts across the country. Fertility programs associated with academic programs and teaching hospitals are also trustworthy.

The situation is even more complicated when patients are
young at the time of the diagnosis and cannot really predict
whether they will one day want to have children or not. It is
important to remind even relatively young patients with cancer that their desire to have children will change as they grow
older and that it is better to keep their fertility options open as
much as possible, even when a discussion about parenthood is
theoretical. Research suggests that many cancer survivors believe that the experience of having cancer will make them bet-

ter parents in the future. But any hope that is given needs to be real and not exaggerated: at the present time, options are limited. However, things may change over time as new techniques are developed.

Brad had his semen tested, and the results were not what they had hoped for. His sperm count was low, and many of the sperm were slow and did not swim as they were supposed to. He was crushed. Brit tried to cheer him up.

"Hey, honey, they can at least swim . . . maybe not that well, but there's still hope, right?"

Brad just looked at her with his big brown eyes. The news had been devastating to him, and he felt like a complete failure as a man. And the irony was that they weren't even thinking about having kids for at least five years after they got married! And now that seemed to be impossible. He knew that Brit wanted a family, so why would she stay with him if he couldn't give her one? He thought about it all the time, and he talked and talked about it. Brit couldn't understand why he kept on and on about it.

"But Brad, can't you let it go for now? We'll worry about that when the time comes and we want to have kids. Can't we just focus on the wedding now and enjoy our time together before the kids come?"

But Brad couldn't let it go. He began to feel like everyone could tell that he was half a man—the guys at work and at the gym. He grew more and more depressed and angry and took most of his bad moods out on Brit. One day she gave him an ultimatum: either he get some help, or she was going to cancel the wedding that was now just six months away.

EFFECTS OF INFERTILITY ON COUPLES AND INDIVIDUALS

Experiencing difficulties with fertility can cause significant stress for many couples. It is common for couples to blame each other for the cause of the problems, even if it is not clear whose "fault" it is. For men and women, infertility can lead to feelings of inadequacy in the male or female role, even though being able to conceive is not what defines us as men and women. In couples dealing with infertility, the rates of depression are twice as high as in couples with no problems. Satisfaction with the relationship and sexual difficulties may result. It is not rare for couples to separate after years of trying unsuccessfully to conceive.

Treatment of infertility also has significant associated costs, which can place additional strain on any couple. For couples where one person wants a baby more than the other, this difference in desire to parent can put additional strain on the relationship. Many fertility clinics insist that couples going through treatment receive a psychological assessment before initiating treatment. Many have social workers and counselors on staff or as consultants to help couples experiencing relationship strain during the often long process of trying to conceive.

Many couples find that trying to make a baby takes all the fun and joy out of sex. Sex becomes a chore that has to be done at a certain time, no matter what else is happening in the relationship or in life. This can cause resentment and even sexual problems if the man feels that he has to perform on demand. Some men develop erectile problems as a result of this pressure.

Having sperm banked has been shown to decrease stress for some men with cancer, as they at least have the hope that one day they can be parents. Some cancer survivors are also worried that they may pass on a genetic predisposition to their children for cancer. However, inherited cancer syndromes account for only 10%–15% of cancers, so this concern is exaggerated. Other survivors are fearful that their treatment may cause birth defects in their babies; this worry is also unwarranted. It is more likely that the long-term and late effects of cancer treatment such as heart or lung problems will cause health risks for the woman when she is pregnant.

Some couples may choose to adopt children instead of pursuing expensive and uncertain fertility treatments. Although not well studied, there are some anecdotal reports that birth mothers reject couples for adoption if there is a history of cancer in one of the potential adoptive parents. Also, some international adoption agencies will not consider couples with a cancer history or will insist on letters from an oncologist stating that the survivor has a normal anticipated life span and has been cancer free for five or more years.

Some people may assume that they are sterile after cancer treatment and may not use contraception when they are sexually active. This may result in unwanted pregnancy and places the individual and partners at risk for sexually transmitted infection if unprotected sex occurs.

Brit hated giving him this ultimatum. She wanted nothing more than to share her life with him, but it was as if he was a different person. She hated seeing him in so much pain. Her mom was a nurse, and even though she worked with orthopedic patients, she knew a lot of people at the hospital and had done some information gathering for Brit. She gave her daughter the name of a fertility clinic in Atlanta, about an hour's drive from where they lived. Brit called and made an appointment, telling Brad about it the weekend before. That sure made him mad, but she told him that he had to go with her, and that if he didn't, it was over.

The drive to the clinic that Wednesday was a quiet one. Brad was still angry that she had made the appointment with the specialist without talking to him, and she was feeling guilty about telling him that their wedding would not happen if he didn't go to the appointment.

But things got better once they arrived. The doctor that they saw was kind and very professional. But more than that, he offered them hope and dispelled much of Brad's pessimism. He told them that his sperm results were not that bad—he had seen way worse—and that there was a procedure where they could take a single sperm and place it directly into one of Brit's eggs. The procedure was called ICSI (intracytoplasmic sperm in-

jection). Although it was expensive, it was widely used in couples where the man has a low sperm count.

Brit grinned as Brad looked up at her, his big brown eyes now filled with hope. She smiled at him and took his hand. The wedding would happen; their life together could begin.

TAKE-HOME MESSAGES

Cancer treatments can affect fertility, but the effects of this may not be seen for many years. Fertility preservation techniques are limited, especially for women, and decisions about this have to be made before treatment starts. This can pose a challenge because the time of diagnosis is a chaotic one. For some individuals, treatment may not be able to be delayed to allow for collection of sperm or eggs. Not all patients or their parents are informed sufficiently to make a decision about fertility preservation, which may mean that the cancer survivor has to deal with regret and suffering years later when trying to conceive a baby. New reproductive technologies offer hope, but they are expensive and not available to everyone, and some do not have great success.

CHAPTER 12

RESOURCES

WEB SITES

The following are some reputable organizations and their Web sites where you can find additional information about cancer survivorship.

- American Cancer Society: www.cancer.org
- Cancer*Care*: www.cancercare.org
- Centers for Disease Control and Prevention: www.cdc.gov/cancer/survivorship
- LIVESTRONG: www.livestrong.org
- National Cancer Institute, Office of Cancer Survivorship: http://dccps.nci.nih.gov/ocs
- National Coalition for Cancer Survivorship: www.canceradvocacy.org
- Oncology Nursing Society's "The Cancer Journey": www.thecancerjourney.org
- Patient Advocate Foundation: www.patientadvocate.org

BOOKS

The following is a list of books on cancer survivorship.

- *After Cancer: A Guide to Your New Life*, by W.S. Harpham, 1995, New York, NY: Harper Paperbacks.

- *The Cancer Survivor's Guide: The Essential Handbook to Life after Cancer*, by M. Feuerstein and P. Findley, 2006, New York, NY: Da Capo Press.
- *Crazy Sexy Cancer Survivor: More Rebellion and Fire for Your Healing Journey*, by K. Carr, 2008, Guilford, CT: Globe Pequot Press.
- *Everyone's Guide to Cancer Survivorship: A Road Map for Better Health*, by E. Rosenbaum, D. Spiegel, P. Fobair, and H. Gautier, 2007, Kansas City, MO: Andrews McMeel.
- *Everything Changes: The Insider's Guide to Cancer in Your 20's and 30's*, by K. Rosenthal, 2009, Hoboken, NJ: John Wiley and Sons.
- *From Cancer Patient to Cancer Survivor: Lost in Transition*, edited by M. Hewitt, S. Greenfield, and E. Stovall, for the Institute of Medicine and the National Research Council of the National Academies, 2006, Washington, DC: National Academies Press.
- *Handbook of Cancer Survivorship*, by M. Feuerstein, 2007, New York, NY: Springer.
- *100 Questions and Answers about Life after Cancer: A Survivor's Guide*, by P. Tolbert and P. Damaskos, 2008, Sudbury, MA: Jones and Bartlett.
- *Picking Up the Pieces: Moving Forward after Surviving Cancer*, by S. Magee and K. Scalzo, 2007, New Brunswick, NJ: Rutgers University Press.
- *What Helped Me Get Through: Cancer Survivors Share Wisdom and Hope*, edited by J. Silver, 2009, Atlanta, GA: American Cancer Society.

MINDFULNESS-BASED STRESS REDUCTION

In Chapter 2, you read about mindfulness-based stress reduction. Many resources are available to help you learn more about this and get you started.

- *Arriving at Your Own Door: 108 Lessons in Mindfulness*, by J. Kabat-Zinn, 2007, New York, NY: Hyperion.
- *Coming to Our Senses: Healing Ourselves and the World Through Mindfulness*, by J. Kabat-Zinn, 2006, New York, NY: Hyperion.
- *Full Catastrophe Living: Using the Wisdom of Your Body and Mind to Face Stress, Pain, and Illness*, by J. Kabat-Zinn, 1990, New York, NY: Delta.
- *Guided Mindfulness Meditation* [CD], by J. Kabat-Zinn, 2005, Louisville, CO: Sounds True.
- *Letting Everything Become Your Teacher: 100 Lessons in Mindfulness*, by J. Kabat-Zinn, 2009, New York, NY: Delta.
- *Mindfulness for Beginners* [CD], by J. Kabat-Zinn, 2006, Louisville, CO: Sounds True.
- *Wherever You Go, There You Are*, by J. Kabat-Zinn, 2005, New York, NY: Hyperion.

SENSUAL MASSAGE AND SENSATE FOCUS EXERCISES

In Chapter 10, a technique was mentioned to help couples get back in touch physically. The following is a detailed description of sensate focus exercises based on sensual massage. Sex therapists and counselors have used this technique successfully for years with couples experiencing sexual challenges.

Sensate focus exercises help to reduce anxiety about sexual performance and increase communication, pleasure, and closeness between couples. When doing sensate focus exercises, each member of the couple takes turns touching the other following the instructions below.

- Decide who will be the first person to do the touching.
- Decide whether you and your partner will be clothed or unclothed; either way is fine.
- Choose where you are going to do this. You both need to be comfortable, and the bedroom may not be the best place.
- You may want to dim the lights and play music you both enjoy.
- Use pillows to support your bodies and keep warm.
- You may use baby oils, scented oils, lotions, or powder if you wish.
- Tell your partner what feels good and what doesn't.
- Start with caressing the face. Normally the person doing the massage (the giver) sits, and the person receiving the massage (the receiver) lies flat on his or her back and rests the head on the other person's thighs. With lubricated hands, if desired, the giver begins with the chin, then strokes upward over the cheeks, forehead, and temples. Then the ear lobes, lips, and the nose are stroked before returning to massage the temples. Stop after about 10 minutes and rest. Talk about the experience and what it felt like for both of you. Then reverse roles.
- Massage the rest of your partner's body and think about what it feels like to be massaged and to do the massaging.

Take turns with major zones of the body—the back, shoulders, and neck; arms and legs; and the abdomen. Genital and breast massage is not included in sensual massage, but you may get carried away!

The goals of this touching exercise are

- To enrich the relationship
- To express your needs and desires in different ways
- To discover how each of you likes to touch and be touched
- To explore new patterns of pleasuring that are not overtly sexual
- To help the relationship grow and change
- To reduce the fear of physical changes.

Sensate Focus Exercises

Sensate focus exercises are similar to sensual massage but they are supposed to be done in a more prescribed manner. The exercises are divided into four stages, and couples are supposed to do each stage before progressing to the next, depending on their comfort.

It is suggested that when you massage your partner that you use your nondominant hand so that the experience feels new to you too. It is important to make the time to do these exercises regularly and to do them when you are well rested and not rushed for time. The aim of these exercises is to explore your feelings and physical sensations of touching and being touched. Sexual intercourse is forbidden, as this is **not** the aim of the exercises. Do not talk while you are doing the exercises; the person receiving the touch can guide the hand of the one doing the massage. You can share your feelings after you are done.

This massage should be done at least three times a week, taking about 20–30 minutes each time (10–15 minutes per person). Take about two to three weeks for each stage before progressing to the next. This requires patience and control, as many couples want to rush to stages three and four.

Stages of Sensate Focus

First stage: Limit touching and stroking to the areas of the body that are not sexually stimulating. Avoid the breasts and genitals.

Second stage: Touch, stroke, and explore the sensual responses of the entire body, including the breasts and genitals without intent to bring about erection or vaginal lubrication.

Third stage: After stroking the whole body as in stage 2, stroke the penis and clitoris and probe the vaginal opening with the finger. Note any physical responses such as an erection or vaginal lubrication.

Fourth stage: Caress and stimulate breasts and genitals after stroking the whole body as in stage 2. Use a lubricant, especially for the clitoris, the outer lips, and the vaginal opening, as well as for the male partner with less than full erectile response. When the man's erection is firm enough to attempt penetration, the couple will want to insert the penis and feel it in the vagina.

If the female feels her partner is losing his erection, she can initiate pelvic movements until it returns. There is no demand for either partner to perform. The exercise is never over as long as the couple feels comfortable with each other and are enjoying and savoring the sensations.

The use of baby oil or body lotion is recommended for stages one and two of the sensate focus exercises. A sexual lubricant is helpful during stages three and four when the genitals are touched.

FERTILITY ORGANIZATIONS

In Chapter 11, you read about a couple facing the challenges of not being able to have a baby after cancer treatment. Many fertility clinics exist across North America, but they may not know about treating cancer survivors. Ideally, any fertility specialist should work with your oncology care provider to provide you with the best care possible based on your own history of cancer treatment.

Some helpful resources include the following.

- **American Society for Reproductive Medicine:** www.asrm.org
  This nonprofit organization ensures that members must demonstrate the high ethical principles of the medical profession, show an interest in infertility, reproductive medicine, and biology, and adhere to the objectives of the society. The Web site contains information specifically for people with cancer.

- **American Fertility Association:** www.theafa.org
  The American Fertility Association is another national nonprofit organization that provides services and materials free of charge including an extensive online library, monthly online webinars, telephone and in-person coaching, a resource directory, an "Ask the Experts" online feature, daily fertility news, and a toll-free support line.

- **Fertile Hope:** www.fertilehope.org
  Fertile Hope is a national LIVESTRONG initiative dedi-

cated to providing reproductive information, support, and hope to patients with cancer and survivors whose medical treatments present the risk of infertility.

BIBLIOGRAPHY

CHAPTER 1

Mullan, F. (1985). Seasons of survival: Reflections of a physician with cancer. *New England Journal of Medicine, 313,* 270–273. doi:10.1056/NEJM198507253130421

President's Cancer Panel. (2004). *President's Cancer Panel 2003–2004 annual report: Living beyond cancer: Finding a new balance.* Bethesda, MD: U.S. Department of Health and Human Services, National Institutes of Health, National Cancer Institute.

CHAPTER 2

Gil, K.M., Mishel, M.H., Belyea, M., Germino, B., Porter, L.S., LaNey, I.C., & Stewart, J. (2004). Triggers of uncertainty about recurrence and long-term treatment side effects in older African American and Caucasian breast cancer survivors. *Oncology Nursing Forum, 31,* 633–639. doi:10.1188/04.ONF.633-639

Mehnert, A., Berg, P., Henrich, G., & Herschbach, P. (2009). Fear of cancer progression and cancer-related intrusive cognitions in breast cancer survivors. *Psycho-Oncology, 18,* 1273–1280. doi:10.1002/pon.1481

Rosedale, M. (2009). Survivor loneliness of women following breast cancer. *Oncology Nursing Forum, 36,* 175–183. doi:10.1188/09.ONF.175-183

Royer, H.R., Phelan, C.H., & Heidrich, S.M. (2009). Older breast cancer survivors' symptom beliefs. *Oncology Nursing Forum, 36,* 463–470. doi:10.1188/09.ONF.463-470

Simard, S., Savard, J., & Ivers, H. (2010). Fear of cancer recurrence: Specific profiles and nature of intrusive thoughts. *Journal of Cancer Survivorship, 4,* 361–371. doi:10.1007/s11764-010-0136-8

Vivar, C.G., Whyte, D.A., & Mcqueen, A. (2010). 'Again': The impact of recurrence on survivors of cancer and family members. *Journal of Clinical Nursing, 19,* 2048–2056. doi:10.1111/j.1365-2702.2009.03145.x

CHAPTER 3

Boyajian, R. (2010). Depression's impact on survival in patients with cancer. *Clinical Journal of Oncology Nursing, 14,* 649–652. doi:10.1188/10.CJON.649-652

Fulcher, C.D., Badger, T., Gunter, A.K., Marrs, J.A., & Reese, J.M. (2008). Putting evidence into practice: Interventions for depression. *Clinical Journal of Oncology Nursing, 12,* 131–140. doi:10.1188/08.CJON.131-140

Pirl, W.F., Greer, J., Temel, J.S., Yeap, B.Y., & Gilman, S.E. (2009). Major depressive disorder in long-term cancer survivors: Analysis of the National Comorbidity Survey Replication. *Journal of Clinical Oncology, 27,* 4130–4134. doi:10.1200/JCO.2008.16.2784

Reich, M. (2008). Depression and cancer: Recent data on clinical issues, research challenges and treatment approaches. *Current Opinion in Oncology, 20,* 353–359. doi:10.1097/CCO.0b013e3282fc734b

Rosedale, M. (2009). Survivor loneliness of women following breast cancer. *Oncology Nursing Forum, 36,* 175–183. doi:10.1188/09.ONF.175-183

CHAPTER 4

Bretibart, W., & Alici, Y. (2008). Pharmacologic treatment options for cancer-related fatigue: Current state of clinical research. *Clinical Journal of Oncology Nursing, 12*(Suppl.), 27–36. doi:10.1188/08.CJON.S2.27-36

Kangas, M., Bovbjerg, D.H., & Montgomery, G.H. (2008). Cancer-related fatigue: A systematic and meta-analytic review of non-pharmacological therapies for cancer patients. *Psychological Bulletin, 134,* 700–741. doi:10.1037/a0012825

Minton, O., Richardson, A., Sharpe, M., Hotopf, M., & Stone, P. (2008). A systematic review and meta-analysis of the pharmacological treatment of cancer-related fatigue. *Journal of the National Cancer Institute, 100,* 1155–1166. doi:10.1093/jnci/djn250

Mitchell, S.A., Beck, S.L., Hood, L.E., Moore, K., & Tanner, E.R. (2007). Putting evidence into practice: Evidence-based interventions for fatigue during and following cancer and its treatment. *Clinical Journal of Oncology Nursing, 11,* 99–113. doi:10.1188/07.CJON.99-113 van der Lee, M.L., & Garssen, B. (2011). Mindfulness-based cognitive therapy reduces chronic cancer-related fatigue: A treatment study. *Psycho-Oncology*. Advance online publication. doi:10.1002/pon.1890

CHAPTER 5

Bellizzi, K.M., Rowland, J.H., Jeffery, D.D., & McNeel, T. (2005). Health behaviors of cancer survivors: Examining opportunities for cancer control intervention. *Journal of Clinical Oncology, 23,* 8884–8893. doi:10.1200/JCO.2005.02.2343

Blanchard, C.M., Courneya, K.S., & Stein, K. (2008). Cancer survivors' adherence to lifestyle behavior recommendations and associations with health-related quality of life: Results from the American Cancer Society's SCS-II. *Journal of Clinical Oncology, 26,* 2198–2204. doi:10.1200/JCO.2007.14.6217

Irwin, M.L., & Mayne, S.T. (2008). Impact of nutrition and exercise on cancer survival. *Cancer Journal, 14,* 435–441. doi:10.1097/PPO.0b013e31818daeee

Kuhn, K.G., Boesen, E., Ross, L., & Johansen, C. (2004). Evaluation and outcome of behavioural changes in the rehabilitation of cancer patients: A review. *European Journal of Cancer, 41,* 216–224. doi:10.1016/j.ejca.2004.09.018

Mayer, D.K., Terrin, N.C., Menon, U., Kreps, G.L., McCance, K., Parsons, S.K., & Mooney, K.H. (2007). Health behaviors in cancer survivors. *Oncology Nursing Forum, 34,* 643–651. doi:10.1188/07.ONF.643-651

Pinto, B.M., & Trunzo, J.J. (2005). Health behaviors during and after a cancer diagnosis. *Cancer, 104*(Supp. 11), 2614–2623. doi:10.1002/cncr.21248

CHAPTER 6

Aziz, N.M., Oeffinger, K.C., Brooks, S., & Turoff, A.J. (2006). Comprehensive long-term follow-up programs for pediatric cancer survivors. *Cancer, 107,* 841–848. doi:10.1002/cncr.22096

Cantrell, M.A., & Conte, T.M. (2009). Between being cured and being healed: The paradox of childhood cancer survivorship. *Qualitative Health Research, 19,* 312–322. doi:10.1177/1049732308330467

Kadan-Lottick, N.S., Robison, L.L., Gurney, J.G., Neglia, J.P., Yasui, Y., Hayashi, R., … Mertens, A.C. (2002). Childhood cancer survivors' knowledge about their past diagnosis and treatment. Childhood Cancer Survivor Study. *JAMA, 287,* 1832–1839. doi:10.1001/jama.287.14.1832

Massimo, L.M., & Caprino, D. (2007). The truly healthy adult survivor of childhood cancer: Inside feelings and behaviors. *Minerva Pediatrica, 59,* 43–47.

Nunez, S.B., Mulrooney, D.A., Laverdiere, C., & Hudson, M.M. (2007). Risk-based health monitoring of childhood cancer survivors: A report from the Children's Oncology Group. *Current Oncology Reports, 9,* 440–452. doi:10.1007/s11912-007-0062-8

CHAPTER 7

Breslau, E.S., Jeffery, D.D., Davis, W.W., Moser, R.P., McNeel, T.S., & Hawley, S. (2010). Cancer screening practices among racially and ethnically diverse breast cancer survivors: Results from the 2001 and 2003 California Health Interview Survey. *Journal of Cancer Survivorship, 4,* 1–14. doi:10.1007/s11764-009-0102-5

Findley, P.A., & Sambamoorthi, U. (2009). Preventive health services and lifestyle practices in cancer survivors: A population health investigation. *Journal of Cancer Survivorship, 3,* 43–58. doi:10.1007/s11764-008-0074-x

Hawkins, N.A., Smith, T., Zhao, L., Rodriguez, J., Berkowitz, Z., & Stein, K.D. (2010). Health-related behavior change after cancer: Results of the American Cancer Society's studies of cancer and survivors (SCS). *Journal of Cancer Survivorship, 4,* 20–32. doi:10.1007/s11764-009-0104-3

CHAPTER 8

Breckenridge, L.M., Bruns, G.L., Todd, B.L., & Feuerstein, M. (2011). Cognitive limitations associated with tamoxifen and aromatase inhibitors in employed breast cancer survivors. *Psycho-Oncology.* Advance online publication. doi:10.1002/pon.1860

Dietrich, J., Monje, M., Wefel, J., & Meyers, C. (2008). Clinical patterns and biological correlates of cognitive dysfunction associated with cancer therapy. *Oncologist, 13,* 1285–1295. doi:10.1634/theoncologist.2008-0130

Nelson, C.J., Nandy, N., & Roth, A.J. (2007). Chemotherapy and cognitive deficits: Mechanisms, findings, and potential interventions. *Palliative and Supportive Care, 5,* 273–280. doi:10.1017/S1478951507000442

Staat, K., & Segatore, M. (2005). The phenomenon of chemo brain. *Clinical Journal of Oncology Nursing, 9,* 713–721. doi:10.1188/05.CJON.713-721

CHAPTER 9

de Boer, A.G.E.M., Taskila, T., Tamminga, S.J., Frings-Dresen, M.H.W., Feuerstein, M., & Verbeek, J.H.A.M. (2010, September). Interventions to enhance return-to-work for cancer patients: A Cochrane review. From the *Proceedings of the First Scientific Conference on Work Disability Prevention and Integration* (p. 86), Angers, France.

Grunfeld, E.A., Rixon, L., Eaton, E., & Cooper, A.F. (2008). The organisational perspective on the return to work of employees following treatment for cancer. *Journal of Occupational Rehabilitation, 18,* 381–388. doi:10.1007/s10926-008-9152-1

Hoffman, B. (2005). Cancer survivors at work: A generation of progress. *CA: A Cancer Journal for Clinicians, 55,* 271–280. doi:10.3322/canjclin.55.5.271

Mehnert, A. (2011). Employment and work-related issues in cancer survivors. *Critical Reviews in Oncology/Hematology, 77,* 109–130. doi:10.1016/j.critrevonc.2010.01.004

Short, P.F., & Vargo, M.M. (2006). Responding to employment concerns of cancer survivors. *Journal of Clinical Oncology, 24,* 5138–5141. doi:10.1200/JCO.2006.06.6316

CHAPTER 10

National Cancer Institute. (2011). Sexuality and reproductive issues (PDQ®). Retrieved from http://www.cancer.gov/cancertopics/pdq/supportive care/sexuality/HealthProfessional

CHAPTER 11

Burns, K.C., Boudreau, C., & Panepinto, J.A. (2006). Attitudes regarding fertility preservation in female adolescent cancer patients. *Journal of Pediatric Hematology/Oncology, 28,* 350–354. doi:10.1097/00043426-200606000-00006

Forman, E.J., Anders, C.K., & Behera, M.A. (2010). A nationwide survey of oncologists regarding treatment-related infertility and fertility preservation in female cancer patients. *Fertility and Sterility, 94,* 1652–1656. doi:10.1016/j.fertnstert.2009.10.008

Quinn, G.P., Vadaparampil, S.T., Lee, J.-H., Jacobsen, P.B., Bepler, G., Lancaster, J., … Albrecht, T.L. (2009). Physician referral for fertility preservation in oncology patients: A national study of practice behaviors. *Journal of Clinical Oncology, 27,* 5952–5957. doi:10.1200/JCO.2009.23.0250

Schover, L.R. (1999). Psychosocial aspects of infertility and decisions about reproduction in young cancer survivors: A review. *Pediatric Blood and Cancer, 33,* 53–59. doi:10.1002/(SICI)1096-911X(199907)33:1<53::AID-MPO10>3.0.CO;2-K

Schover, L.R., Brey, K., Lichtin, A., Lipshultz, L.I., & Jeha, S. (2002). Knowledge and experience regarding cancer, infertility, and sperm banking in younger male survivors. *Journal of Clinical Oncology, 20,* 1880–1889. doi:10.1200/JCO.2002.07.175

Schover, L.R., Brey, K., Lichtin, A., Lipshultz, L.I., & Jeha, S. (2002). Oncologists' attitudes and practices regarding banking sperm before cancer treatment. *Journal of Clinical Oncology, 20,* 1890–1897. doi:10.1200/JCO.2002.07.174

van den Berg, H., & Langeveld, N.E. (2008). Parental knowledge of fertility in male childhood cancer survivors. *Psycho-Oncology, 17,* 287–291. doi:10.1002/pon.1248

INDEX

A

acute effects, 118
acute survival, 2
alcohol use, 89, 91, 97
   avoidance of, 67, 71, 87
   as coping method, 19
   and smoking, 84
alkylating agents, 118
American Association of Sexuality Educators, Counselors, and Therapists (AASECT), 174, 175
American Society for Reproductive Medicine, 191, 192, 205
Americans with Disabilities Act, 154–155
amputation, 115, 151, 163
androgen deprivation therapy (ADT), 119, 163, 165
antidepressants, 48, 49, 52, 67, 86, 139
anxiety, 15–18, 21
   in childhood cancer survivors, 106
   and chronic pain, 57
   and cognitive changes, 127, 129, 131
   and mindfulness-based stress reduction, 24
   and progressive muscle relaxation, 51
   and return to work, 152
   and sensate focus exercises, 202
   and sexual pain, 175
   and support groups, 30
aromatase inhibitors, 112, 130, 166
arousal, 163, 164, 173

B

back-to-work plan, 10. *See also* work
bisphosphonates, 123
body image, 7, 115, 116, 162, 163, 180
breast cancer
   and cognitive changes, 129–130, 139
   and lifestyle changes, 122
   and loneliness in survivors, 40
   risk of, with alcohol use, 87
   and sexual issues, 166, 172, 174
   support groups, 29

C

cancer free, 2, 6, 195
cancer survivorship
   definitions of, 1–4
   seasons of, 2

carcinogens, 122
cardiovascular disease, 116, 119,
    121, 123
chemobrain, 10, 127
chemo fog. *See* chemobrain
chemotherapy
    in childhood cancer survivors,
        104
    and cognitive changes, 127–129
    and depression, 46
    and exercise, 79
    and fatigue, 53, 56, 57
    and fertility effects, 183–185
    long-term and late effects of,
        111–112, 114, 118–119,
        121, 124
    and post-traumatic stress disor-
        der, 43
    and sexual changes, 165, 180
    and survivorship care plan, 93,
        97
childhood cancer, 104–108
cisplatin, 118
cognitive-behavioral therapy
        (CBT), 45, 46, 52, 59, 140
colon cancer, 55, 99, 111, 164
colonoscopy, 122
colorectal cancer, 116, 122
complementary therapies, 51, 88
crisis intervention, 46
cryopreservative, 189
cyclophosphamide, 118
cytokines, 57, 56, 129

D

deep breathing, 23, 24, 32
denial, 19, 40
dental caries, 124
dental problems, 111, 117, 121
depression, 9, 33–35, 39–41, 111,
    116
    and cognitive changes, 127, 129,
        140

and exercise, 26, 64
and fatigue, 56–57, 59, 69, 91
and infertility, 194
and return to work, 152
and survivorship care plan, 99
de-professionalizing, 37
diabetes, 10, 72, 109, 116, 118,
    119, 121, 123
diarrhea, 111, 117
diary, 20, 137
diet, 65, 69, 71–75, 77, 88, 89, 97,
    99, 122, 124
discrimination, 154, 155, 159
    in the workplace, 143, 149, 154,
        155, 159
drug use, as coping method, 19

E

egg freezing, 189
embryo freezing. *See* egg freezing
endocrine therapy, 97, 112
end of treatment, 2, 5, 6, 37
energy conservation, 61
estrogen, 128, 129, 130, 139, 165,
    166, 172, 174, 175
exercise, 9, 26, 32, 50–52, 59–60,
    64, 69, 71, 78–83, 89, 91,
    97, 115, 123, 141
extended survival, 2
external cues, 15

F

faith-based practice, 28
Family and Medical Leave Act
        (FMLA), 155, 156
fatigue, 7, 9, 18, 53–57
    and cognitive changes, 131, 141
    and depression, 35, 37
    and exercise, 91
    interventions for, 59–62, 64–69
    and lack of sexual desire, 164

as long-term/late effect, 109, 111, 119
and return to work, 151, 153, 159
and smoking cessation, 86
fatigue scale, 60
fear, 7, 8, 9, 13, 14, 16–21, 23, 26, 31, 32, 35, 90, 115, 139, 165, 169, 187, 203
Fertile Hope, 189, 205
fertility preservation, 187, 189, 197
forgetfulness, 131, 137
From Cancer Patient to Cancer Survivor: Lost in Transition, 96, 200

H

head and neck cancer, 87, 147
hormonal changes, 163, 165, 175
hormone-dependent cancers, 189
hormone therapy, 128
hot flashes, 10, 116, 119, 136

I

immune suppression, 110, 119
infertility, 11, 114, 194, 205, 206
insomnia, 54
Institute of Medicine, 96, 200
internal cues, 14
intrusive thoughts, 16, 20, 21, 32

J

Journey Forward, 102

L

label reading (nutrition information), 75
Leydig cells, 185

LHRH agonists. *See* luteinizing hormone-releasing hormone (LHRH) agonists
libido, 119, 164, 165, 166, 172
lifestyle changes, 9, 57, 89
LIVESTRONG, 102, 199, 205
lubricants, 174, 204
luteinizing hormone-releasing hormone (LHRH) agonists, 130
lymphedema, 117, 163

M

massage therapy, 51, 62, 69
masturbation, 179, 188
menopause, 112, 115, 118, 127, 185
menstrual cycle, 112, 185, 189
methotrexate, 118, 119
methylphenidate (Ritalin®), 139
mindfulness-based stress reduction (MBSR), 23–26, 32, 201
motivation, 9, 51, 59, 79, 82, 83, 86, 89
multiagent chemotherapy, 118
music, 83, 202

N

National Cancer Institute, 3, 86, 199
National Comprehensive Cancer Network, 102
neutral zone, 6
nutrition, 56, 64, 65, 69, 71, 73–78

O

obesity, 65, 72
Office of Cancer Survivorship, 3, 199
orchiectomy, 116
organic food, 76, 77

orgasms, 115, 163, 165, 174, 179
osteoporosis, 10, 88, 112, 121, 123
ostomy, 116
ovum, 185

P

pain, 14
  emotional, 52
  and fatigue, 56, 57
  as long-term/late effect, 111,
      114–115, 116, 118–119
  and mindfulness-based stress
      reduction, 24–26
  and return to work, 152
  and sexual problems, 163–166,
      171, 173, 175
Pap smears, 122
post-traumatic stress disorder
    (PTSD), 43–45
Prescription for Living, 102
President's Cancer Panel, 3
progressive muscle relaxation, 21,
    25, 32, 51
prostate cancer, 111, 115, 130, 162,
    163, 165, 167, 172, 176, 179

R

radiation, 37
  and childhood cancer survivors,
      104–106
  and cognitive changes, 129
  effects on fertility, 183–185, 190
  and exercise, 79
  and fatigue, 53
  long-term/late effects of, 109–
      111, 114, 116–117, 119,
      121, 123, 124
  and post-traumatic stress disor-
      der, 43
  and sexual problems, 165–166,
      180

and survivorship care plan, 97
rehabilitation programs, 82, 157
relationship changes, 10
Ritalin®. *See* methylphenidate

S

saturated fat, 74, 75
secondary cancers, 2, 3, 9, 87, 105,
      116, 118, 121
sensate focus exercises, 171, 175,
      201, 202, 203, 204
sensual massage, 201, 203
sex, and the single person, 179
sexual desire, 116, 118, 164, 166,
      172
sexual dysfunction, 116, 119, 161,
      162–166
  barriers to treatment for, 177–
      178
  interventions for, 170–176
  talking about, 168
sexuality, 8, 11, 99, 161, 164, 167,
      174, 177, 178, 180, 211
side effects
  late effects, 3, 14, 97, 98, 105,
      106, 109, 113, 114, 116,
      118, 121, 122, 124, 125, 195
  long-term, 7, 10, 53, 79, 97, 98,
      105, 109, 111, 112, 119,
      124, 164, 195
skin cancer, 87, 117
sleep, 34, 35, 42–44, 46, 48, 49, 53,
      54, 57, 64, 66, 67, 69, 116,
      130, 131, 136, 139, 141, 153
smoking, 71, 84–86, 89, 97, 123
sperm banking, 187, 188, 212
steroids, 112, 118, 119
sun protection, 71, 87, 91
super foods, 76
supplements, 88
support groups, 29, 30–32, 84
  for smoking cessation, 86
surgery, 37, 93

and cognitive changes, 129
effects on fertility, 183–185
and fatigue, 53
for fertility preservation, 190
long-term/late effects of, 111,
  113–116
nerve sparing, 177
pelvic, 114
reconstructive, 14
and sexual effects, 162–165, 170,
  179, 180
and survivorship care plan, 97
survivorship care plan (SCP), 10,
  48, 96–102, 108, 125

T

talk therapy, 46
testosterone, 116, 118, 119, 129,
  130, 163, 165, 166, 172, 175
transitional cancer survivorship, 2
transplantation, bone marrow and
  stem cell, 3, 46, 112

U

urinary problems, 111
U.S. Department of Agriculture
  food guidelines, 77

V

vitamins, 76, 88, 99, 123

W

work
  discrimination, 154–155
  interferences with, 109, 115, 143
  medical leave, 155–156
  return to, 54, 145–159
written reminders, 137

Y

yoga, 23, 25, 50, 82

ALSO FROM ANNE KATZ

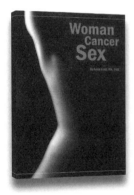

WOMAN CANCER SEX

A. Katz

"The perfect book for healthcare providers as well. I can't strongly enough recommend that you keep the book in an obvious place. Even if a patient never talks to you about sex, seeing the book in your office will give them permission to go home and order it from Amazon. If books were to get grades, this one would earn an A or an A+, and I'm not an easy grader."—Paul Joannides, Psy.D., author of *Guide to Getting It On*, winner of the AASECT Book Award for 2009

2009. 184 pages. Softcover.

Retail Price: $14.95

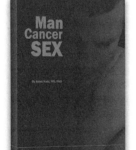

MAN CANCER SEX

A. Katz

In a follow-up to her popular book *Woman Cancer Sex* (see above), Dr. Anne Katz explores how men are affected by a diagnosis of cancer and how they can seek help. Each chapter describes the experience of men with various types of cancer and the problems they may face, including pain, loss of libido, erectile dysfunction, fertility challenges, and more.

Written for men and the women (and men) who love them and live with them through their cancer journey, *Man Cancer Sex* is a book that men can read to help them understand their situation and communicate openly with their partner.

2010. 176 pages. Softcover.

Retail Price: $19.95

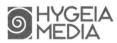

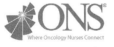